ADOLESCENT IMMATURITY
Prevention and Treatment

Publication Number 873

AMERICAN LECTURE SERIES®

A Monograph in

The BANNERSTONE DIVISION *of*
AMERICAN LECTURES IN LIVING CHEMISTRY

Edited by

I. NEWTON KUGELMASS, M.D., Ph.D., Sc.D.

Consultant to the Departments of Health and Hospitals
New York, New York

ADOLESCENT IMMATURITY

Prevention and Treatment

By

I. NEWTON KUGELMASS, M.D., Ph.D., Sc.D.

Consultant to the Departments of Health and Hospitals, New York; Heckscher Institute for Child Health, New York; Osteopathic Hospital, New York; Lynn Memorial Hospital, Sussex; Monmouth Memorial Hospital, Long Branch; Muhlenberg Hospital, Plainfield; Northwoods Sanatarium, Saranac; Honorary Pediatrician, Misercordia Hospital, New York.

Formerly, Exchange Scholar from Johns Hopkins University; Instructor in Chemistry, Columbia University; Professor of Chemistry, Samford University, Birmingham; Pediatric Research Associate, Yale University Medical School; Director Pediatric Research, Fifth Avenue Hospital; Attending Pediatrician, French Hospital; Hospital for Ruptured and Crippled; Riverside Hospital; Manhattan General Hospital; New York City Children's Hospital.

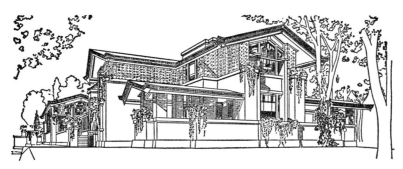

CHARLES C THOMAS • PUBLISHER

Springfield • Illinois • U.S.A.

Published and Distributed Throughout the World by

CHARLES C THOMAS • PUBLISHER

BANNERSTONE HOUSE

301-327 East Lawrence Avenue, Springfield, Illinois, U.S.A.

© *1973, by* CHARLES C THOMAS • PUBLISHER

ISBN 0-398-02707-2

Library of Congress Catalog Card Number: 72-88449

With THOMAS BOOKS *careful attention is given to all details of
manufacturing and design. It is the Publisher's desire to present books
that are satisfactory as to their physical qualities and artistic possibilities
and appropriate for their particular use.* THOMAS BOOKS *will be true
to those laws of quality that assure a good name and good will.*

Printed in the United States of America

JJ-V

Hail, blooming Tacee!
Given so much of Earth,
So much of Heaven,
To create aspirations, dreams.

FOREWORD

Our Living Chemistry Series was conceived by Editor and Publisher to advance the newer knowledge of chemical medicine in the cause of clinical practice. The interdependence of chemistry and medicine is so great that physicians are turning to chemistry, and chemists to medicine in order to understand the underlying basis of life processes in health and disease. Once chemical truths, proofs, and convictions become foundations for clinical phenomenon, key hybrid investigators clarify the bewildering panorama of biochemical progress for application in everyday practice, stimulation of experimental research, and extension of postgraduate instruction. Each of our monographs thus unravels the chemical mechanisms and clinical management of many diseases that have remained relatively static in the minds of medical men for three thousand years. Our new Series is charged with the *nisus élan* of chemical wisdom, supreme in choice of international authors, optimal in standards of chemical scholarship, provocative in imagination for experimental research, comprehensive in discussions of scientific medicine, and authoritative in chemical perspective of human disorders.

Dr. Kugelmass of New York fuses the scientific and the compassionate in the evaluation and interpretation of the immature adolescent for early prevention and individualized treatment. The adolescent is a growing and becoming creature singularly adaptable to almost any environment in the struggle for maturity. Identity predominates but genetic diversity maintains at the expense of biologically inferior organisms that are inadequate, weak, and sick. The difference between a mature and an immature adolescent at any age level is somewhat like the difference between a tooth and a stone—the one is highly organized and the other is not; the one is highly integrated and the other is not; the one is highly functional and the other is not. Each bears physical and chemical patterns but the stone is just a confusion.

It is only when life appears that you begin to get organization on a large scale; life takes the atoms and molecules and crystals, combines them into elaborate patterns of its own, instead of making a mess of them like the stone. The confusion so deeply rooted in the adolescent immaturities finds expression in malfunction while the confusion in his internal struggles finds expression in misbehavior until reversed by adequate and balanced maturation. Life's great objective during adolescence is to form optimal patterns for optimal integration for optimal maturation.

The normal adolescent is a labile organism with wondrous diversity in behavior, in motivation, in response to stress, in virtually every function he is called upon to perform. What a cunning mixture of sentiment, pity, tenderness, irony surrounds youth. But teen-agers with innate incapacity, inadequate rearing, or excessive stress become unequal to the challenges of everyday life in form and/or function. They are the maladaptive, the immature, the handicapped, the sick in body and mind—physically, mentally, emotionally, socially, and sexually—that need guided parental protection, individualized medical care, and specific psychiatric concern. The scientific view of the adolescent must thus be fused with the compassionate. There is no clinician truly great and generous who is not also tender and compassionate. He sees youth as a full-fledged member of society who thinks, feels, believes, wants, remembers, struggles, and loves. He sees him as a fascinating, terrible, and lonely being, desperate, gregarious, passionate, and cruel. He sees him as a person who feels pity as a learned emotion, who laughs, who has a sense of humor. All of this and more is gleaned from the author's subjective introduction in the Preface for the more objective approach integrated for individual application in everyday practice, whatever the degree of adolescent immaturity.

> "And youth is cruel and has no remorse
> And smiles at situations it cannot see."

THE EDITOR

PREFACE

"Let each become all that he was created capable of being; expand, if possible, to his full growth; resisting all impediments, casting off all noxious intrusions, and show himself at length in his own shape and stature, be these what they may."

Every clinician concerned with the growth and development of children heeds Carlyle's counsel to help immature adolescents achieve optimal maturity. It is not enough to take steps which lead to the goal; each step must be itself a goal and step likewise, to enter the ripe and fertile season of action when alone youth can hope to find the head to contrive and the hand to execute. It is much easier to go from one childhood to another than to pass the turbulent arena between childhood and adulthood, from immature love with peace to unstable passion without peace, from carefree oblivion to knowing watchfulness, from rainbow raiment to Zodiac bravery, from the passive to active voice, from latent strength to manifest manhood that survives all worldly hurt.

Adolescent growth is a last leap in the dark, a spontaneous, unpremeditated act without benefit of experience that transforms an immortal child into a mortal youth, who parts with faith and his love against his will to renew the faith and recreate the passion. But the hypothalamic clock triggers the internal revolution irreversibly. It is as natural a growth as an oak. It comes out of the past. Its foundations are laid far back. It is the most powerful human force to break the parental fetters and build an independent life-style. It is the daring search for freedom and self-fulfillment of youth. Inferiors revolt that they may be equal and equals that they may be superior; so much of adolescence is an ill-defined dying, an intolerable waiting, a longing for another place and time, another condition.

The problems of adolescents are always the same but the solutions are ever individual. No problem of human destiny is beyond youth. There is no developmental deviate, no matter what his measured intelligence, distorted physique, impaired function, unstable emotion, inadequate sex, meager sociality, unbalanced personality may be, who is beyond significant increments of functional and adaptive improvement. Unfortunately, the picture is obscured by anxiety which impairs abstract and associative thinking, saps free energy, vitiates constructive motivation, distorts perception, suppresses learning behavior, and decreases effective functioning. In this age of anxiety, the age of the neurosis, so much weighs on youths' minds and even more grates on their nerves.

Anxiety and conscience are a powerful pair of dynamos; between them they ensure that youth shall work hard, but they cannot ensure they shall work at anything worthwhile. The feeling of youth's own dignity is achieved only through work and struggle. When the work is a pleasure, his life is a joy; when a duty, his life is slavery. To be what he is, is the first step toward becoming better than he is. Constraint from without and freedom from within are two aspects of the same necessity, the necessity of being the person he is and not another. He is free to be that individual, but not free to be another.

Adolescence is not an end but a means. The means prepares the end, and the end is what the means have made it. The journey from means to end may be long and tedious but the means themselves are enjoyed if the end is ardently desired. It should be rounded development of an integrating personality performing physical and mental work, creating material and spiritual values, and evolving a personal philosophy of life. We must take the larger view of immature youth, that potentially great responses already exist inside him and that these responses need only to be catalyzed to become manifest. We must behold youth as infinitely malleable, infinitely perfectable, infinitely capricious, and as a privilege to guide and treat such towering possibilities.

Youth is the time to do something and be somebody. It is like a fruit tree that is not yet productive but symbolizes the beauty of a growing personality and anticipates its glorious future. It reflects the genetic background and the consummate care provided by parent, teacher, doctor and society. It is from the first fruits they bear that we learn what may be expected in the future. It is a turbulent period of body transformation into the real self, a struggle for independence from parental domination, an adjustment to the world in quest of harmonious sex, occupation and sociality. It is the crystallization of a fruitful philosophy of life to answer, What am I? What ought I to be? What may I hope? What can I believe? Youth labels its ignorance and calls it knowledge, but time and experience alter his perspectives.

Every diagnostic evaluation illuminates how we can aid immature adolescents to attain the fullest substantive growth and functional performance possible—physical, intellectual, emotional, sexual, and social, all integrated into a unique nobody in a world which is doing its best, day and night, to make him everybody else. Early recognition of developmental deviation is the business of the parent even more than of the physician, hence an adolescent immature for his age may wear a wrong diagnosis around his neck like a millstone. The doctor's primary task is to un-diagnose him to get at the core of the problem and avoid being mousetrapped by tangential data. He will for a time dismember the patient scientifically to isolate the dynamic components of his being, but in the end put them together again in his final diagnosis for the total conception of the interrelationships between the adolescent as a person, the disorder as part of the patient, and the patient as part of the world in which he lives.

When an adolescent is weighed in the clinical balances and found wanting, the development deficits must be determined promptly and treated effectively. The immature patterns are evaluated in seven chapters according to the developmental, physical, mental, emotional, sexual, social, and personality defects, deviations, and disorders respectively. We may dissect youth into these systems but we must not be led astray by such divisions, for human thought, feeling, and action are holistic, not segmental. Then too it is difficult to make asymptomatic youth feel better, for the course of correction is too slow to satisfy, ever complicated by primary and secondary disorders precipitated by exacting tasks that may lead to chronic ailments at maturity. We are particularly concerned with functional problems: recurrent headaches, refractive errors, hearing loss, ugly acne; with structural problems: obesity, thyroid nodules, spinal curvatures, short stature, excessive tallness; with digestive disorders: peptic ulcer, ulcerative colitis; with sexual problems: masturbation, gonadal status, breast changes, menstrual disorders, sex relations; with heredofamilial problems: hypertension, bronchial asthma, rheumatic fever, tuberculosis, diabetes, and renal disorders. The physician has two sleeves, one containing a diagnostic and the other a therapeutic armamentarium; both sleeves should rarely be emptied in one move. Some techniques should be kept in reserve and the maneuvers turned to best serve the changing status and special needs of the adolescent. The earnest desire to succeed by all concerned is almost always prognostic of success; and the secret of adolescent success is constancy to purpose.

The global upsurge of medical concern with the shape of things to come is the first tentative answer to the challenge of the vast new forces man has freed by research and development. He is now compelled to fashion scientific techniques to enable him to exert fuller control over his powerful material tools. It is a stage in the evolution of humanity, an important step towards medical maturity to advance the adolescent cause. The future is no more uncertain than the present; study of the future will bring us nearer to the day when man will be able to choose desirable futures and shape rather than suffer his destiny. And so I have added an epilogue on Adolescence 2000 envisioning adolescent, medical and community advances respectively. Yesterday is not youth's to recover, but tomorrow is his to win.

I.N.K.

MEANING

The word "he" throughout the text refers to boy or girl according to Old English and American tradition. Every word in the language was at first a stroke of genius. Every word was once a poem. Each began as a picture. Somehow the structure of language remains relatively static so that the unceasing changes of man and the world can be interpreted. If meanings changed as quickly as events, no event would have a meaning. When the living language in which we think and have our being becomes depraved, it is followed by degradation. Only in Genesis was the whole Earth of one language and of one speech. To grasp the meaning of the world today we use a language created to express the world of yesterday. The life of the past seems to us nearer our true natures, but only for the reason that it is nearer our language. The meaning of words lies not in the words themselves but in our attitude towards them. Indeed, meaning receives its dignity from words instead of giving it to them.

ACKNOWLEDGMENTS

My first and well-nigh inexpressible indebtedness goes to teen-age patients who cooperated year after year to unravel the underlying basis of their deep-seated disorders in order to formulate the developmental concepts of adolescent immaturities; to deeply concerned parents of troubled teen-agers who revealed so much from thoughts and feelings about paradoxes of experience with their raw progeny, that harbored seeds of new conceptions about maturation; to friends and colleagues in American, European, and Asian Universities for the intellectual spurs of fruitful discussions and thoughtful communications that enabled reduction of so vast a field to reasonable compass.

I am grateful to Mr. Joseph Anthony Vario for collecting and cataloguing the significant bibliography. The vast clinical and experimental literature covers so many disciplines to supply the answers to adolescent immaturities that we must resort to choice rather than to exclusion. To give chapter and verse for every statement between these covers would be a formidable task indeed, while references to only the most recent papers would serve little useful purpose at a time when progress is so rapid in all adolescent fields. I have therefore adhered to the policy adopted in similar works and given only recent review articles and books, since the bulk of research reported herein has occurred in this generation. These I believe can serve either to expand the general reader's horizons or provide starting points for a more intensive study of particular fields.

Finally, I wish to express my warm gratitude to Miss Virginia Chaffin-Schmidt for indispensable secretarial services; to Miss Ruth Georgia Beck for constructive criticism of the manuscript and precise proofreading; to Mrs. Rachael Peck Gartner for meticulous typing and for preparing a good index; to my devoted publishers, particularly Mr. Payne Thomas and Mr. Robert Schinneer and their diligent staffs, not only for the excellence of their craftsmanship, which speaks for itself in these pages, but also for their wholehearted cooperation in every way and at every stage of the production of every monograph of our Living Chemistry Series.

CONTENTS

Contents

ADOLESCENT IMMATURITY
Prevention and Treatment

CHAPTER I

DEVELOPMENTAL IMMATURITY

Nature does not require that we be perfect;
It requires only that we grow, and we can do
this as well from a mistake as from a success.

One of the assets of youth is to feel incomplete; and the overwhelming truth about youth is that it is incomplete. It requires no apology, for in incompleteness there is promise, because the adolescent is not merely unfinished but self-fabricating by his will to form. He is, as it were, the leopard who knows how to change his spots, the creature who has the secret of becoming what he wills. Instead of taking his life as it comes and adapting himself to external conditions, he is constantly evaluating, discriminating, choosing, reforming, and transforming at every moment of his existence to achieve his independent SOS, e.g. sexuality, occupation, sociality with variety, for anything that promises variety or seeks change has youth. The paradox of youth is desire for stability but need for change to soothe his troubled soul; he confronts the paradoxical but exposes himself to reality with pubescence, an act of Nature and to adolescence, an act of man.

Adolescent development involves values when the directed change produces tangible growth; a growing apple passes through a sequence of stages, and one stage is best; we reject green and rotten apples and accept ripe ones. Farmers work to bring crops safely to maturity; and parents, teachers, and doctors strive to produce mature adults. Positive changes in the direction of maturity reveal becoming, while negative changes in delayed, arrested, or defective development, being immature. Man arrives at morphological maturity at about twenty-two years to remain on this plateau of reasonable stability with a thousand voices in rebuke of youth. Even the mature individual can continue to develop long after most grown-ups have muffled themselves in the cocoon of adult convention. Maturity becomes a

3

goal, and progress becomes movement toward a goal, a terminus that is temporal, not spatial. It is not enough to take the steps towards a goal; each step must be itself a goal and a step likewise. A windmill is eternally at work to accomplish one goal although it shifts with every variation of the weathercock, like an adolescent, and assumes ten different positions in a day to attain the endless goal.

The drama of adolescent life is like a puppet show in which stage, scenery, actor, and all are made of the same stuff. The players have their exits and their entrances but the exit is by way of transition into the substance of the stage; and each entrance is a transformation scene. So stage and players are bound together in the close partnership of an intimate comedy; and if we would catch the spirit of the piece, our attention must not at all be absorbed in the characters alone, but must be extended also to the scene, of which they are borne, on which they play their part, and with which, in a little while, they merge again. The great and glorious masterpiece of man is to know how to live to purpose, and the secret of adolescent success is constancy of purpose.

Lack of Maturation Fulfillment

Contemporary forces are creating a new kind of protean adolescent in psychological flux throughout his maturation changes. Even the styles of inner stability differ from time to time. There is no model youth to portray all happenings for inner revolutionary forces are ever dislocating the outer identity of youth. The self is his symbol of his being and the self-process his psychic recreation of that symbol in flux. It is as natural a growth as an oak; it comes out of the past; its foundations are deep-seated in the immature metabolism. Proteus in Greek mythology readily changed to many forms but resisted a single form. That's the current feeling of protean youth—polymorphous versatility of a subjective mind in action for confrontation with objective forces. Adolescent life without such absorbing activity is hell; joy consists in forgetting life. The moment youth is on the side of life, peace and security drop out of consciousness. The only peace, the only security is in fulfillment. But youth lacks the ideology that can give coherence to his world without a sense of symbolic integrity. Music must know discord to produce harmony; medicine must know disease to produce health; adolescence must know immaturity to produce maturity. Youth's immaturity is but imbalance without wisdom for masterful administration of the unforeseen.

Adolescent immaturity is in unstable equilibrium in all systems of the organism. It is charged with free energy readily accessible for the dynamic processes of multiple maturation, the end stage of stored entropy. Thermodynamics is the unique science to establish relations between different forms of body energy which allow us to peep behind the inner scenes of youth's workshop. Free energy flows from transfer reactions in which unsaturated bonds are transferred from one molecule to another by enzyme catalysis. It is the adolescent energy of total immaturity that stirs the exciting feature of creative thought, the exhilarating feelings for new living, the aberrant behavior for impulsive expression. All is perpetrated by shrinking from the responsibility of standing and acting alone. And the irresponsibility is measured not by the amount of injury dissipated from wrong action but by the distinctness with which conscience can distinguish between the right and the wrong.

Adolescents are immature without being aware of it. The developmental process in the making is an art to be learned, an effort to be sustained in striving for maturity; the ripe season of action, when alone youth can hope to find the head to contrive, united with the hand to execute. Yet the unstable period of inadequacy clears spontaneously with dynamic growth unto maturity. In the interim there is immaturity in structure and function of body and mind, sociality and sex, emotionality and spirit. And each immaturity has its own level, adding to the incongruity of the unintegrated personality in the making. Multiple immaturity complicates the course, effectiveness, and fulfillment of maturation for the enrichment of one system is without effect on other systems.

Physical inadequacy slows growth; mental inadequacy curtails learning; emotional inadequacy distorts feeling; social inadequacy bars independence; sexual inadequacy precludes fulfillment; spiritual inadequacy blocks transcendence. All are living processes surging forth vectorially unto the resultant maturity. Youth is not the arithmetical sum of what he has already at any stage of adolescence but rather the sum of what he does not yet have, of what he could have.

Lack of Self-transforming Capacity

The problems of immaturity are always the same but the solutions differ with each adolescent, projected from dependence to independence, from subordination to dominance, from sexual neutrality to mature control. This drastic transformation in life is the only art adolescents are required to practice without being allowed the preliminary trials, the failings, the botches that are so essential for the training of a mere beginner. But the art of life is to know how to enjoy a little and endure a lot so as to give a meaning and a value of his own to life. The adolescent veers between Scylla and Charybdis balancing the centripetal force that holds him back in the easy family realm and the centrifugal force driving him into the difficult world arena. Youth must seize the opportunity to do something and become somebody in his season of hope, enterprise, and energy. Almost everything that is great has been and will be done by youth because youth is wholly experimental. Only by passing through the fire of experiment will the adolescent become a purposefully acting adult fulfilling the two standards of maturity: the ability to love and the ability to work.

Can the adolescent be modified? Of course he can. Is he not changed by everything that happens to him in everyday life? Youth of today does not differ essentially from the one who lived in the caves a hundred thousand years ago. Man's history which has gone by since that age has scarcely altered the morphological and physiological being. Indeed, if it were possible to place an adolescent of that past age into our own time and rear and educate him as one of ours, he would become an individual exactly like us, an individual who nothing, either in appearance, or in his conduct, or in his private thoughts, would be singled out as a stranger among us, as a ghost from the past. He would meet with no difficulty in initiating himself into the complexity of our customs about to resist, rebel and revolt as well as anybody else. After all, man is at bottom an animal, midway a citizen, and at top divine; but the climate of this world hasn't changed since antiquity, hence few ripen at the top.

The current problem is to change the adolescent's inherent possibilities, produce a fresh organic change in him, develop a taller, or more robust, or more virulent, or more handsome being; more intelligent, more clever, sensitive, more disposed to solidarity and altruism to be more human. A man thinks, feels, loves, suffers and admires with the whole of his being and with all of his organs. A mature man achieves genital primacy. The genitalia become the center of libidinal excitation, and the pregenital-component instincts are subordinated to genital primacy or sublimated. It is the genital primacy that enables man to achieve instinctual pleasure and to function within a cycle of excitation, or tension, and discharge at pleasure. This basic cyclical patterning becomes an aspect of character. He can work and rest, give conscious and sustained attention to matters of immediate concern, alternate activity with passivity. Youth becomes man only by intelligence, but he is man only by the heart. Hormones reinforce his intellectual power and character; androgens make him more virulent and courageous; estrogens excite the maternal instincts; specific chemical compounds affect social behavior through kindness and devotion; nutrition advances adolescent maturity. The great masterpiece of man is to learn how to live to purpose—optimal in body and mind.

Lack of Unitary Individuality

Man's body and brain have not changed significantly during the past hundred thousand years. Physiological functions still undergo cyclic changes linked to the cosmic forces of evolution. We still operate with the physiological equipment that fitted us to the natural environment of the late Stone Age. All human beings have the same anatomical structure, operate the same physiological processes, exhibit the same biological urges, yet no two are alike at any time, through all time. Every individual is unique and every adolescent develops his own behavioral singularity. Some mechanisms of individuality have their roots in the evolutionary past; some, in the genetic endowment; and others, in the environmental responses. Genes do not determine traits but only govern the responses of the individual to environmental stimuli. Individuality is as much a product of the total environment as of the genetic endowment; it can thus be regarded as the incarnation of the response that the organism has made to the influences that have impinged on it throughout development.

The epoch of individuality is being concluded, and it is the duty of the reformers to initiate the epoch of association. Collective man is becoming omnipotent upon the earth he treads, abstracting individuality from its citizenry and making the individual an abstraction. Everything without tells the individual he is nothing; everything within persuades him that he is everything. What mammoth differential between outer and inner forces for youth; what insurmountable task to overcome; what tremendous potential to grade into equilibria between the outer world and the inner man. How can there be an enlightened state if the state fails to recognize the individual as an independent power from which all its own power is derived and not treat him accordingly.

The greatest works are done by the individual; the hundreds do not often do much; the companies never. It is the units, the single individuals, that are the power and the might. Individual effort is, after all, the grand thing to cultivate through individual development. Individuality is inherent in every being from conception to dissolution in the physical structures, chemical processes, and physiological arrangements that mediate this determination. What is bred in the bone must come out in the flesh.

Modern medicine, too, suppresses the recognition of individuality in computer diagnosis and treatment. The disturbing problem of individual diversity has been submerged under an extravagant technical curriculum to the detriment of maturity in the making and will remain so until medicine wakes up to its full obligations to genetic youth with respect for individuality.

Once youth has realized that he carries the world's fortune in himself and that a limitless future stretches before him in which he cannot flounder, his first reflex may lead him along the dangerous course of seeking fulfillment in isolation. Some innate instinct stirs him to break away from the crowd to find the utmost limit of himself, but he becomes retrograde in such isolation. To become fully himself is in the opposite direction, in the direction of convergence, with all the rest; he must advance toward the others. The peak of his self is not his individuality but his person. He can only find his person by uniting together from top to bottom. There is no mind, no growth, no maturation without synthesis. The true ego varies inversely with egoism. He must not confuse his individuality with his personality. He must identify, harness, and develop his intercentric nature to evolve as a unitary individual among all others in his daily realm.

The biochemical individuality is like an iceberg with most of its manifestations submerged and only a small part visible to the examiner. We have reason to believe that everyone is a deviate potentially, important enough for understanding the slight disorders that impede full maturation. The rate of maturation is accelerated by improvement in nutrition, by control of infection, by balance of body hormones, by increase of heterosis through the wide range in the choice of a mate that leads to hybrid vigor. Man is programmed by the caliber of intrauterine and postnatal life over which he has no control. He can never change his past for all manifestations of his free will are delineated by this early patterning. The most that society can do is to provide conditions so diversified that each person has multiple opportunities for obtaining the necessary and sufficient materials of life. The modern world will thus be as favorable to the expression of individual development and biological freedom as the most advanced periods in the history of mankind, provided all potential abilities are cultivated. All that is valuable in human society depends upon the opportunity for development accorded to the maturing individual.

Genes determine potential strength of any inherent ability, but they do not guarantee their expression. Each gene manifestation is regulated by chemical feedback from the environment and from the products of other genes to produce adaptability for greater fulfillment. Youth will be successful if the power of accommodation is equal to the strain of fusing continuous internal and external changes. Every developmental system of the body can be taken apart and put together to study the interactions of the component cells and tissues in evaluating the caliber of maturation in the making. Once the integrative factors that control such interactions are known, we will bridge the gap between studies of development at the whole organism level with those at the molecular level, and then trace the pathway from the action of the gene in youth to the final expression of its phenotype at maturity. The developmental process represents an integration of constitutional and learned changes in the adolescent makeup. Change implies a transition from the state of another while development focuses upon a one-directional component of change. Development is a dynamic process; change, an end-product. Normal development depends upon predictable change at definite constancy in change while deviant development is nonproductive in both rate and intensity of organic growth and sociopsychological maturation.

The developmental theory of Gesell, the cognitive theory of Piaget, the learning theory of Sears and the psychological theory of Erikson together present an associated frame of reference for adolescent development. All aspects of adolescent life are considered as so many facets of a unitary integrated individual rather than artificial components of separate disciplines. Understanding the depth and breadth of an adolescent's development is a prerequisite for effective work with deviated development in body, affect, cognition and behavior. The adolescent has a particular predisposition for creating internal conflict and anxiety. His massive neocortex provides the potential for learning fine discriminations of complex social cues and for anticipating danger in the absence of immediate stimuli. But the visceral brain which holds the neocortex tends toward mass response with less discrimination, producing dangerous effects throughout the organism. The inhibitions acquired during childhood bring these mass reactions and reverberating internal feedback that precipitate needless stress throughout youth. It is a period of anxiety and neurosis because much weighs on his mind and so much more grates on his nerves.

The adolescent's pattern of psychosocial dependence does not necessarily parallel his maturational tempo. Adolescence is a time for exploration, for vocational planning, for choosing a dating companion, for accepting one out many philosophies of life. Each youth must be dealt with as an individual rather than as a representative of an age or sex group or as a person typed by any aspect of his behavior. We know far more than we apply. It takes a systematic understanding of the individual to implement helping tasks more knowingly and more creatively once his status has been established. Individual development is never fully completed or entirely normal in an adolescent's life. Few adolescents will develop physically in every system according to my clinical experience; few will develop cognitively in all ways according to Piaget; few will successfully resolve all affective conflicts according to Erikson's modal phases; few will achieve full satisfaction or tension reduction from every goal-directed response according to Sears' phases.

Lack of Maturing Criteria

All systems of the adolescent organism cannot achieve complete internal and external equilibria to form a balanced personality equal to the challenges of maturity. Youth is only geared for the physical and mental, not for the emotional and social requisites of love and work. Any differential between chronological age and physical, mental and emotional maturation leads to latent or active psychiatric disturbance. And, inadequate emotional and social development for the age level play havoc not only with balanced maturation processes but with adult independence attainment. Asynchronous development of the total personality is thus the forerunner of unsuspected maladjustment for a lifetime as long as society fails to facilitate normal maturation en masse. Where, when, who, what and how is immaturity? Where refers to the geographic location; when, to the time factors involved; who, to the individual characteristics; what, to the definition and classification; how, to the method of observing. The ultimate question is why immaturity?

Immaturity indications in early childhood are early warning signals for detecting latent adolescent problems; disturbances in eating, eliminating and sleeping displace adaptive equilibria during stress; pica and cyclic vomiting reflect severe physiologic or psychologic stress; colic and insomnia produce possible CNS immaturity arising from the mother's inability to nurture the infant. Delayed development is evident from marked retardation in curiosity at five months, vocalization at six months, hand investigation at eight months, verbalization at one year, and sphincter control at fifteen months. A serious problem indicator is the loss of previously acquired skills from illness, injury, or alienation from the mother. Continued over-reaction to mild stress, repeated impulsiveness, intolerance of frustration are critical indicators of personality difficulty. Early recognition of immaturity is the business of the parents even more than of the physician.

Immaturity forewarnings in the school child are school vomiting, school phobia, temper tantrums, impulsive activity, and asocial withdrawal. The hyperactive youngster who creates school turmoil may veer towards subsequent delinquency. Difficult transitions from class to class or teacher to teacher bespeak emotional difficulties generated by unstable parents. Nervous system instability, greater in boys than in girls, points to potential problems in speech, learning and reading. Overt symptoms of home and school difficulty expose the child as the most vulnerable member of the family constellation. The mother is the best thermometer but the child is the obvious sufferer—avoiding school, troublesome, stammering, failing peer relations, and committing antisocial acts.

Immaturity manifestations in the puberal child from increased stress is revealed by self-doubt, sudden changes in behavior, refusal to undress in the gymnasium, and persistent masturbation. The suffering of the adolescent is evident in his withdrawal from friends and family, in school phobias, learning difficulties, and inexplicable violence. Such odd behavior may well mark the beginning of acute psychosis or the threat of suicide and homicide. Persistence of such manifestations requires prompt evaluation of the adolescent, his family and school setting and appropriate intervention to correct the abnormal situation for reducing future disability. A misleading manifestation is misleading only to one able to be misled; the sound clinician attacks the core of the problem and avoids being mousetrapped by tangential data.

The universal danger of parental optimism that cumulative problems will fade away constitutes wishful feeling and that the difficulties will be outgrown reflects primitive thinking. The facts are that prolonged stress from any cause whatsoever before the third year of life may lead to irreversible CNS damage that interferes with the child's innate capacity to learn things first hand, to develop sensory-motor skills, to proceed along the stepping stones of increased physical functioning, to achieve a real sense of personal competence, to become outgoing in relations with others. Every latent or blatant handicap must be assessed at the onset in early childhood, curbed effectively, observed for complication and treated accordingly. The personality in the making crystallized at adolescence becomes delimited by the weakest manifestation in the link. The great objective is for the physical, mental, emotional and social assets of youth to be synchronized for optimal health for optimal maturation for optimal independence.

Lack of Parental Understanding

Every generation revolts against the parents but makes friends with the grandparents. Parents' brains shrink while youths' brains swell. Parents use their brains so little when it comes to their omnificent adolescents that when they do, it is only to make excuses for their reflexes and their instincts, only to make their crude acts appear more studied. Parental reactions to adolescent sexuality play havoc with youth. Sexual maturation takes the family by surprise as an unexpected event; the childhood manifestations of the sexual impulses are disregarded or deprecated, and the successive puberal events are ignored or confirmed in the privacy of the bedroom in some families and/or shared as achievements by others. Hostile reactions to maturity contrast with the overflow of tenderness to immaturity, much to the bewilderment of youth.

The transition from the asexual adolescent puts parental psychosexual maturity to the test. The object of overt love during childhood becomes a sexual stimulating taboo in adolescence. It reactivates their own adolescent struggles with overt autoerotic homosexual and oedipus conflicts to the development of adolescent decompensation in retrospect. Families have two crises in their midst: the adolescent crisis in the child and the reactivity crisis in the parents. In the underprivileged, one-third of the illegitimate pregnancies are the products of incestuous union, mainly with the father. It is the characteristic of the father with near incestation relationships with his daughter to react to adult heterosexual interest on the part of the girl with prudish indignation. Sexual rivalry in the family creates disruptive effects on marriage; a daughter may become a serious rival to a mother who has been thwarting the husband for years even though adolescent sexuality becomes a stimulus to parental sexuality.

Adult reactions to adolescent maladjustment aggravates home misery. Adults and teachers assume that the great emotional upheaval produces bizarre personal changes convincing the adolescent of the justification for his swings in moods and waywardness. But the overall picture does not simulate psychiatric illness. Healthy adolescents may have psychotic symptoms such as anxiety, depression, complexes or phobias; character difficulties such as excessive sensitivity, attachment rigidity, intellectualization and perfectionism. Psychological deviations tend to be single rather than multiple, mild in intensity, and episodic without impairing function. Such fluctuations demand parental flexibility. It is not easy to shift comfortably with emotional swings since youth is unaware of the underlying basis of his misery or happiness. A transient depression may be due to scholastic or vocational difficulty, love affair setback, nostalgia for childhood, or deep-seated introspection. The parental dilemma is aggravated by the adolescent feeling that all adults are his natural enemies.

Adults envy adolescents. Envy is like a fly that passes the body's sound parts and dwells upon sores. Parental envy is stirred by reactions in adolescents—hatred, ambivalence, sadomasochism, jealousy, resentment, reproachfulness, and martyrdom. The basic metabolic distinction between adult and adolescent is vectorial direction; the adult is on the way down and the adolescent is on the way up. The envy may show itself in contrast, derision of remaining adult assets, criticism of youth's awkwardness, and lack of experience in worldly affairs. A father who has done everything better than the son can hardly acknowledge that the son is excelling. One parent will retire gracefully from the scene but another will try to outdo his rival in athletics, even to the point of a coronary attack. Conflict of the generations is civil war and in all such contentions, triumphs over youth are long-range defects.

Parental reaction to adolescent weaning from the family is deep-seated depression. Parents experience a sense of emptiness about the home—a separation of souls, and an absence of lifelong goals. Some family-conscious parents are unable to acknowledge this irreversible loss, attempt to adopt adolescent ways of life, keep pace with youth, but the disguise is evident to the adolescent. Some prevent the escape of the adolescent by enslaving him with incestuous enthrallment which prolongs dependence indefinitely; the parents truly possess the child and block his entrance into adolescence. The ambivalence in the fixation is severe, the pathological immaturity of the child extreme, and the conservation forces destructive to both. A better way of retaining part of the lost childhood is to partake in the process of separation and accelerate the individualization to its total fulfillment. A new relationship thus becomes possible in which the adults are linked by mutually happy memories with many interests in common and new mature pleasures in each other as independent beings. Satisfaction is no longer derived from old anaclitic models but from the rediscovery of the child as an independent adult, provided the parent has relinquished the child at the start of adolescence. But the parent must always remain the lifeguard ever ready in case youth gets beyond his depth.

Lack of World Awareness

The sensibility of youth to trifles and insensibility to great things indicates a strange inversion characteristic of immaturity. No wonder the man of the world arranges his face each morning in order that no one can suspect he has any feeling for anything or anybody. The awakened youth is the one most imbued with the spirit of the time—the impressionable youth. His eyes and ears can see and hear more, his memory can recall at once the impressions of the senses, his imagination can weave a theory of the events. Only that day dawns to which youth is awake. The art of awareness is the art of learning how to make up to the eternal miracle of life with its limitless possibilities. It is developing the deep sensitivity through which youth may suffer and know tragedy and die a little, but through which he will also experience the grandeur of human life. It is learning to interpret the thoughts, feelings, and moods of others through their words, tones, inflections, expressions and movements. It is keeping mentally alert to all that goes on around him to build the great fund of knowledge of the universe. It blocks blind spots in solving problems by striving to see life steadily and see it whole. It is enlarging the scope of his life through the expansion of his personality.

The process of maturity requires dual awareness of being an observer and participant in the world. Youth can harmonize the search for meaning with the search for an adult role in society. His commitment to exploration in sex, sociality, communal living, politics indicates that the whole being is being organized into a new personality. Youth born into a closed cultural pattern, whose members have strong social superegos, has no urge to transform into a new being and there is no adolescent rebellion. But youth in our cultural systems has a feeble sense of relatedness and lives the life of a spider in suspense in a state of semiawareness. He looks for the truth in everything and finds it. He loses faith in the meaning of existence. He revolts against all traditions. He reveals meaninglessness in behavior patterns. He goes on psychodelic trips to enlarge consciousness. He resents adult display of the prevailing hedonism of life with a sense of value based upon purposeless gaining and spending wealth. On the canvas of current history we observe existential philosophy in the West, social deprivation in the developing nations, and historical awareness in Communist societies. Thoughtful youth evolves a new style of life by disintegrating negative values and reintegrating the positive in his way. He cannot mature in a nonexistent psychosocial moratorium and so turns to a socio-existential moratorium to create a new communal superego. Such actions challenge life in Afro-Asian youth, economics in Russia, China and in Israel, and humanities in the West. Such evolution proceeds by jumps in each year; a generation in form and shape can thus achieve what centuries failed to achieve with form.

Lack of Adolescent Termination

Youth has a feeling of eternity which makes amends for everything. To be young is to behave like an immortal supported by technologic, economic, and social evolution that conspire to prolong the dependence of youth upon their elders. It excludes them from the many privileges and responsibilities of adult life by juvenilizing them. Erikson condones the prolongation of adolescence as a triumph of civilization to postpone commitments for social roles while searching for identity. But adolescent irresponsibility is contradictory to the increasing pressure on youth for early occupational planning to know whither they are bound. Obviously, prolonged identity play and selective occupational choice cannot be encouraged simultaneously without conflict. Yet the search for identity serves as a substitute for occupational orientation while coping with problems of sex, education, and vocation. Achieving a stable sense of personal identity provides the adolescent with orienting concepts of the kind of person he is, his strengths and limitations, and his ways of evoking responses.

It is built on a well-established sense of his sex role and his capacity to perform and experience pleasure without guilt. It includes the ability to accept and reject identities that society seeks to impose on the adolescent. Shakespeare's Polonius cautioned his son, "Neither a borrower nor a lender be." A sense of identity can neither be borrowed nor loaned without injuring the adolescent's secure knowledge of who he is, to himself and to his world. Polonius also advised, "This above all—to thine own self be true." Such orientation concepts crystallize into relatively permanent self-attitudes to provide a durable feeling of self-sameness and self-certainty in the face of widely varying life experiences and markedly contrasting relationships. But youth must relinquish his self-image and his childhood role before he is able to fully embrace the adult role. He must give up and even rebel against his dependent relationship to his parents in order to establish a healthy personal identity of his own while maintaining mutual respect to secure parental support. In the interim, he assimilates and experiences growing sexual impulses to reduce his inner tensions while making himself acceptable to his peers without incurring the wrath of adults. Conflicting demands of adolescence make it normal to behave in an unpredictable manner: to fight impulses and accept them, to love parents and hate them, to revolt against them and be dependent upon them, to be ashamed to acknowledge parents and yet desire heart to heart talks with them, to thrive on imitation of and identification with others while searching for personal identity, to be more idealistic, artistic and unselfish and yet be self-centered, egocentric and calculating. The adult structure of personality is thus difficult to crystallize while the ego experiments. Nevertheless, the stresses of adolescence stir exuberance, on the one hand, and loneliness, on the other, throughout this period of turmoil.

Acute identity confusion develops with parental hold on the immature adolescent thwarting normal transitions in relationship. He does not know who or what he is, develops a sense of unreality, a feeling of isolation, a loss of drive, and an inability to adjust to life. The effort to cope with stress leads to the kind of aberrant behavior that reveals negative identity. If prolonged, endless adolescence leads to immaturity as a lifelong phenomenon manifest in various systems of the body with imbalances in the mental, physical, emotional and/or social potentials. The wisdom of the body exacts an harmonious balance of each of these forces, well integrated, to make a truly wholesome personality in the making, but imbalance in developmental tempos creates progressive personality disorders. Body homeostasis attempts to compensate for such imbalances but when the deviations become marked, the personality reflects blatant failure. Youth is pulling in his horse as he is leaping. We must bear in mind that an individual is a thing before he becomes a person. The thing is an integral part of the family or institution or society, while a person has his own objectives. The gradual transition to late adolescence may veer to success via constructive rebellion or unsuccessful failure revealed by each apathetic resignation. Life never presents youth with anything which may not be looked upon as a fresh starting point no less than as a termination. Indeed, the place which seems like the end may also be only the beginning of another venture in the seasons of life.

DEVELOPMENTAL MATURATION

The book of Genesis gives us the four signs of healthy adolescence: desire for knowledge, questioning of authority, realization of sex, acceptance of work. The word is a lamp unto the feet and a light unto the path. Yet the adolescent persists in his childish way of living in the Garden of Eden without the burden of responsibility, without the embarrassment of sex, and above all, without the urge to work. Sooner or later he must leave the Garden to find the prospect gloomy if he remains immature in body, mind or spirit and/or his preparation has been inadequate, misleading or frightening. The crisis is represented in Chinese by the characters danger and opportunity. But the uncertainty may make him attempt to retrace his steps, even though the inevitable course of his life is leading him further from the Garden. Yearning inwardly for the only safe haven he has known, he creates the bizarre manifestations of adolescence disorders. Nevertheless, the exciting thing about adolescent boys and girls is their idealism, free to formulate ideal plans before settling down into disillusionment.

Genetic Controls

Human growth is self-stabilizing or target-seeking with trajectories governed not only by the control systems of genetic constitution but by the energy absorbed from the natural environment. If a child is deflected from its natural growth, trajected by acute malnutrition or hormonal deficiency, a restoring force develops, providing the missing nutrients or hormones to catch up to his original growth curve. When it gets there, growth slows to adjust its path onto the old trajectory once more. The question is how the child knows that it reaches its old trajectory and when to slow down. During the catch-up period the whole organism grows rapidly in a proportionate manner. A systemic stimulus to induce catching up circulates in the blood to all parts of the body to achieve the requisite in size, not in shape. The shape in the human is little affected by a slowdown and the subsequent catch-up in growth. Different effects of malnutrition on the trunk and limbs may occur but not strikingly, since growth in shape is regulated by peripheral rather than by the central mechanism for size.

The catch-up stimulus involves a balance of several hormones released or coordinated by the pituitary in response to a signal which indicates the degree of mismatch between the actual size of the organism and the size required at that age by the larger growth curve. As the target growth curve is approached, maturation diminishes, and the catch-up slows down. The mismatching is a peripheral phenomenon that occurs in all cells and all tissues, each cell carrying the code of its own maturity. Target size regulation is controlled in the brain from conception or three months thereafter when the mechanism begins to function. This tally can represent the target curve, for both are signals made against the continuing time base. The actual height or size of the organism is determined by the concentration of the circulating substance produced by the cells as an inevitable accompaniment of protein synthesis proportional to the size of the organism. The tally represents the maturation rate for each individual organ. The rate of tally, the rate of change of that rate, is ever individual by inheritance. The enzyme systems with reduced activity during the growth period show increased activity after maturity, and conversely those enzymes that have high activity in early life have reduced activity in adult years. Biochemical age can thus be controlled by levels of enzyme activity via nutritional regimen. Biochemical immaturity is amenable to genetic and to environmental factors, for growth and maturity are affected by sex-regulated differences, drug effects, hormones, nutrition, stress, and disease.

Cognitive development proceeds to full ability to use abstract symbols and to think hypothetically and deductively. The period of formal operations begins at eleven years and ends at sixteen years for the development of thinking. It allows the young adolescent to put himself in the place of others and to comprehend their points of view. Moral judgments become more abstract and universal in contrast with childish concrete ideas about right and wrong. Indeed, it is the first time in life that youth senses the true meaning of the abstract forces that bind human relationships—love, charity, empathy, justice and the like. Morality

begins to emerge from democratic rules based on inner conviction, not on the need to please others or to placate authority.
Somehow, youth is least resigned to the way it has to live of
all other living things in creation. And the resistance to parents,
revolt against authority, and rebellion towards the world builds
to turbulent and tumultuous proportions. Some traverse this
period evenly with gradual evolution to maturity, others succeed
only after a tortured passage, but most range somewhere between
these extremes.

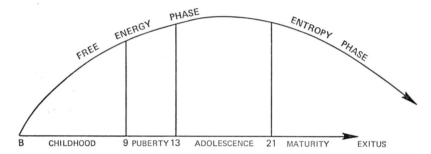

Figure 1. The human trajectory from conception to exitus—adolescence is
the final growth period for completing and/or correcting developmental
needs during the anabolic free-energy phase of youth before the onset of
the catabolic entropy phase of adulthood.

Developmental Cycles

All development is a leap in the dark, a spontaneous unpremeditated act without benefit of experience. It is the human
trajectory pursuing three 6-year growth cycles in the upward
surge of the three developmental stages: sensory-motor, operational thinking, and formal thinking, respectively. The rapid
physical growth in infancy is followed by slower emotional growth
in the preschool period; the rapid mental growth during second
dentition is followed by the slower social growth during school
years; the rapid sexual growth in puberty is followed by the
slower cognitive growth in adolescence. The resulting being is
adequate and balanced if childhood has been effective and com-

plete. Then and only then can youth be thrust out of the finished cycles of life, a leap most difficult to make when he prefers to renew the faith and recreate the passion rather than part with his faith and his love. Some adolescents seem as if they could never have been children, while others seem as if they could never be anything else.

Most adolescents meet the final challenge in the face of danger, but failure to resolve the crisis from young adulthood to advanced age leads to psychiatric problems. The three normal phases of adulthood are alloplastic to acquire mastery over the external world; autoplastic to achieve self-mastery; and omniplastic to help master society. The adult who fails in the struggle gets fixated at the stage that has not been successfully negotiated, makes futile attempts to top the cycle, or retreats to the earlier phase for comfort. The home is the pilot laboratory for the world crises encountered in everyday life. The art of facing reality is cultivated at home, but the science of solving problems is perfected in the real world. A person's development bears the essence of happiness in coping with life if molded by achievements and admiration, and of unhappiness if molded by hostilities and frustrations.

Clearly, there is neither a chronological age nor an actual adolescence of maturation significance. The archaic concept of age must give way to seasons of life which are ever individual because of the wide ranges of each maturation period throughout life. In reality, there are a series of adolescences: the first during the second two decades of life; the second during the next two decades; the third during the subsequent two decades, and so on, each according to individual propensities. Total maturation is a continuous process approached by halfway fulfillments in succession without ever achieving man's full potential. Life is an open system but maturity is a closed one with directional development. Maturation refers to processes of growth which occur relatively independently of the environment; development refers to the interaction between maturational processes and environmental influences which lead to higher structuralization and to individual variations in the human apparatus; and development of the personality refers to the unfolding of the innate constitution under the influence of the changing environment.

Every adolescent must have a solid home foundation to withstand the stresses of the outer world. The foundation, like that of a building, institution or nation, is never seen but is felt when the bearer acts under stress. Then and only then does the caliber of being become transparent. There is a foundation for the stability of the body machine and there is a foundation for the adaptability of the body self. The former provides optimal resistance in coping with the onslaught of adolescent disorders, and the latter in adjusting to the exacting rigors of the world. The body machine is better understood than the adolescent self. One's own self is well hidden from one's self; of all mines of treasure, one's own is the last to be dug up. Its composition is discerned from the onset of emotional stress or from a provocative incident in the youth's milieu, from the circumstances that heighten or lower his feelings, from the form of his relationship with people, from his day dreams or night dreams, from his resistance to transforming insight into action.

The first adolescence is but a continuum of a growing "machinery" charged with free energy and a developing "self" integrating into a unique personality before rising entropy becomes manifest. It may come to pass with deficiency or defect as immaturity for life, apparent only as a complex of diverse levels of underfunctioning, or less often, as poor health in the failing integrity of various functions. Adolescent life is more than permutations in the DNA molecule, just as the Fifth Symphony is more than vibrating air. And adolescent immaturity is more than an aggregate of errors in the adequacy and/or balance of the body machine for the balanced self. It is a universal human experience which has a salvage function in maintaining the vital balance. Perfect development of the body machine, in the sense that every organ gets exactly what it needs for optimal function, is as rare as perfect health; and optimal development of the individual self, in the sense that every latent ability gets what it requires

for maximum cultivation, is as rare as perfect conduct. Maturation is like a chain with all essential components as separate
links; if the chain is weak or broken at any point, the whole chain
fails, hence deficiency or defect in any component leads to immaturity. This concept of adolescent immaturity is relatively new.
It is true that certain developmental deficiencies have long been
recognized as the result of a lack of essential components. These
are gross deficiencies, but new is the concept of immaturity due
to a deficiency of substances or processes which are required
for maturation in minimal amounts. There is genetic anatomical
and biochemical deviation in the adolescent with tissue depletion,
followed in succession by biochemical lesions, functional changes,
and finally anatomic lesions. No step in this chain of events is
necessarily complete before the next begins. Organic disorders
occur in 20 percent of adolescents and functional disorders in 80
percent, hence immaturity may be acute or chronic, mild or
severe, reversible or irreversible, depending on the velocity, intensity and duration of the lesion.

The behavior of cells, tissues and organs of the organism as
a whole is a continuous attempt to preserve, enhance and transcend organic integrity at the everchanging levels of life by adjustments to disturbed balance. The steady state is not only
applicable to the body machine but to the personal self and even
to the environment in which it moves. Changes in the balance
of one system reverberate throughout that system to affect the
steadiness of other systems. Organismic self-regulation strives
for balance by reconciliation of all body demands whereby optimal
satisfaction is achieved at minimal cost and maximum development with least effort. Balance in development is manifest as
polarity, as lines of force, as tensions. The whole organism begets
polarities within itself and these beget tensions, although tension from free energy in cells produces the polarities in the first
place, giving birth to them out of itself. The organization of tension becomes the basic technique in projecting the developmental
tempo. The pattern of tensions reflects subjective feeling orig-
inating within the body like the felt activity of muscles and the

stirring of emotions. Adolescent stability is but balance, and wisdom lies in masterful administration of the unforeseen.

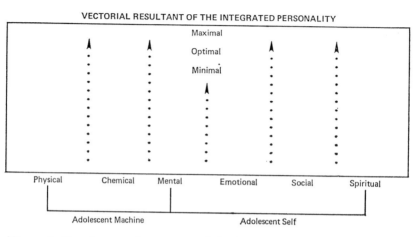

Figure 2. Developmental processes of the body machine and the individual self, essential for maturation—complete if all systems are adequate and balanced, and incomplete if one or more components in any system remain defective, deficient or disordered at maturity.

Maturing Indicators

The adolescent is ambivalent for he knows not who he is, what he stands for, and how much he will stand for. He is a mobile target for objectivity, changes kaleidoscopically and, therefore, is impossible to predict. He may show a precocious sense of morality in the fall and violate all his principles in the spring. He is a kind of inkblot, a projective test for the adult world. Things move so fast for him internally and externally that there is no apparent problem of adjustment to the outsider. Before he can adjust to A, B has appeared leading C by the hand, and D in the distance. He must find ways of keeping his sights on tomorrow, else he cannot be expected to keep in touch with today. The boundless colorful mutability of maturity in the making is enthralling. Childhood is like a fruit tree producing fascinating transformations through growth processes, but adolescence is a cultural fabrication for personal experimentation. Boys and girls become biologically puberal before the culture ascribes the adolescent role to them. Physiological functions, however, become optimal in performance at respective chronological ages and gradually decline in total maturation, cardiac output, vital capacity, muscle strength, heat production, blood flow, and nitrogen excretion. There are many physiological ages in each individual depending on the physiological system evaluated, and there are many maturation indicators to predict growth: skeletal maturity, permanent dentition, radiological evidence of jaw calcification, secondary sexual characteristics, 17-ketosteroid excretion, menarche after the maximum growth velocity and toward the end of puberty.

Maximal attainment of physiological functions at specific chronological ages is identified as maturity with termination of growth. Some physiological functions reach their maximal level at various times after cessation of physical growth, and so no specific chronological age span can be assigned to growth. Many physiological characteristics related to body size are equated in terms of surface area. But an index of total functioning protoplasm in terms of ^{40}K content of body water now offers a better criterion than surface area. Physiological functions reach maturity at different periods in the life cycle: for example, glomerular filtration rate attains adult values at age two years, but blood pressure continues to rise throughout life. If maturity is envisioned as maximum functioning, those functions which fall short of a systemic maximum can never meet such criteria. The concept of physical age is of little value because no unit of measure has been defined. Even when deviation in the age of a child occurs for a specific event, such as the menarche, external time is the unit of measurement, not physiological age. The variability is reduced when individuals are grouped by similarity in size and growth rather than chronological age alone. Nevertheless, growth in different functions can best be described clinically in terms of chronological age.

The prediction of growth from estimates of skeletal maturation indicate the need of early, average, and late maturers for separate standards of growth. Skeletal maturity age is not necessarily related to chronological age in health. Most children closely approximate the common mean curve for weight and height at stated ages. Early maturing children who are taller than average fall moderately above the mean curves but will not become tall adults. But, early maturing children who are genetically taller than average mature rapidly and reach adult status early as tall individuals. Late maturers with or without genetic shortness naturally fall below the average to varying degrees. Unsuspected growth changes in some children may occur suddenly, before expected, or may remain delayed.

Maturing indicators in dentition, in secondary sexual characteristics and in 17-ketosteroid excretion must be correlated for significant deductions. Permanent dentition and skeletal maturation are closely related to the onset of the adolescent spurt, but skeletal maturity is more closely related to puberty than to chronological age. The girl is about two years more advanced than the boy in nearly all maturation indicators at some time in the whole picture of dentition, skeletal maturation, and growth spurt. There is the general maturity advance in the female so common in all mammals, but the place of the genetic factor on the Y-chromosome is not yet established. The menarche usually occurs after the maximal growth velocity and towards the end of puberty but it does not usher in puberty. When a girl of eleven years has not started her puberty or has not menstruated yet, the family becomes alarmed lest she become a "giant." Most of these girls are early maturers with early breast enlargement. They are well along in the accelerated curve of growth velocity and will grow very little more as confirmed by radiological assessment of nearly closed epiphyses.

Body-Mind Ubiquity

Adolescent maturity begins with the prepuberal period manifest by a sharp increase in general body growth, enlargement of the genital organs, change in body configuration with the development of the secondary sex characteristics, appearance of menstruation in the female and ejaculation in the male, emergence of the capacity for the highest form of abstract thinking and reasoning. Libido is concentrated in most of the body changes, particularly in the sexual parts. Even the greatest mental capacity is highly libidinized. There is an actual increase in total energy available, with a resultant strengthening of the sexual and aggressive drives that pose the threat of inadequate impulse control. The changes in body size and configuration disturb the body-image concept that needs to be revised.

The sexual changes provide adult sex functioning and the biologic changes necessary to make him master of himself. The rapid increase in energy and activity is looked upon by society with mixed feelings. Normally, youth is given greater responsibility, but expected to control his sexual impulses subject to adult authority. Aggression is mobilized by frustrations as the adolescent seeks to fulfill his adult destiny under society's controls. A certain amount of rebellion is inevitable and the rest gradually channeled into constructive attempts to gain independence via competitive activity and individual productivity. Increased sexual drives make youth withdraw from parental to peer relationships in conflict with society. Youth often finds satisfactory entente with adults younger than his parents to the point of hero worship. If the hero is a good leader, socially responsible, the adolescent is led in the right direction, but the wrong kind of hero may lead to antisocial behavior. Once the adolescent masters the biological cultural challenges, he again draws closer to his parents. A boy becomes an adult two years before parents think he does, and about two years after he thinks he does.

Increased aggressive drives reawaken the conflicts of childhood. The id-ego-superego equilibrium which had attained a fair degree of stability in the latency stage is upset by the ego to gain mastery over the disturbing forces of adolescence. At times, the ego is in alliance with the superego, and its impulses inhibited to the point of asceticism. At other times, the superego is ignored, and indiscriminate urges are permitted immediate satisfaction. Once the adolescent comes to terms with his new social and aggressive capacities, the psychic equilibrium is reinstated with attainment of a reasonably stable identity which permits pursuit of educational and occupational goals. The increased capacity for self-evaluation and introspection leads to understanding of self. Withdrawal from dependency on the parents weakens the superego derived largely from them. It enables youth to examine many of the value judgments put forth by his parents, select those consonant with his own, and eventually return to the parental pattern of value system. Changing needs in early adolescence create feelings of internal disorganization concealed by bravado and expansiveness, hence the impulsiveness and unpredictability. Intense interest in the peer group is expressed by clothing fads, teenage heroes, and bizarre music.

Personal identity is gradually delineated in adolescence. It provides orienting concepts of strengths and limitations, gives feelings of self-sameness and self-certainty in the face of heterogeneous experience, relinquishes self-images of childhood, assimilates powerful sexual impulses and strong peer affinities. Behavior is unpredictable but normal in fighting impulses and accepting them, loving parents and hating them, and imitating others while seeking self-identity. The concept of body image is revised continuously because his body feels strange to him. Any apparent deviation plays havoc with him, causing loss of self-esteem, agonizing self-consciousness, and unwholesome adaptation when sexual development is atypical in terms of stature, configuration, breast variation, and penis size.

Criticism of self is obstructive; of society, destructive. Adolescents rebel because society appears sick; people are engaged in meaningless work directed toward meaningless wealth; and ritualistic schools impose authority for its own ends. Some gifted adolescents create their own life style; some become activists in social, political, industrial and/or religious realms to save the corrupt world; some withdraw completely from the adult world to create a hippie culture; some are more helpless and escape into the "enchanting world" of drugs. Yet all imitate the adult world in cars, sports, clothes, and even in deficient intellectual pursuits, obscuring similarities with dirtiness, slovenliness, and carelessness. The hippie satisfies psychological needs via communal love—pervasive and undifferentiated, the antithesis of individualism and isolation in society. All communal relations are between the person and the community, not with another person.

Communal enclaves are families of rebellious adolescents enjoying the unspeakable peace and freedom of being orphans. They limit their interaction with adult society, impose intense discipline, destroy the individual self. But the shift of responsibility from the self to the commune provides a psychological extension of the self to eradicate social isolation and its inherent terror. True security is found in social solidarity rather than in isolated effort. All joys are collective, all sorrows diffused. There is freedom from responsibility and continuity of carefree feelings of childhood—blatant immaturity. The whole being enters into all relations, not segments of the adolescent as in dealing with the outer world. Such communal enclaves will become transitional organizations between home and society to provide sociopsychological needs currently unfulfilled. The faithful in the Catholic Church always have the benefit of spiritual care by the Holy Family. Adolescent alienation from society can be circumvented by the development of institutions for satisfying youth's needs as apprentices while performing services and/or undergoing training for independent roles in our industrial society.

Senseless Suffering

"Were we to imagine ourselves suspended in timeless space over an abyss out of which the sounds of revolving earth rose to our ears, we would hear naught but an elemental roar of youth." So said Daetigus centuries ago. Adolescent suffering is man-made. It is not due to the harshness of the elements but to harshness of his fellowmen, mother, father, brother, sister, and to his own reflexive rather than reflective response to these. Much of the perceived harshness is due to inadequate or disordered communication, rectified by orderly or therapeutic or genuine communication. Ideal communication is clear-cut and congruent, intended to be mutually beneficial, respects the integrity of both participants, accepts the limitations and tolerates the defects of both.

Adolescents suffer; they bear up or endure with distress, with body pain, and with mental grief from the stress of maturation. Suffering is the sole price of a more searching vision; otherwise, his gaze of life must be shallow and without intellectual revelation. He never reasons so much and becomes so introspective as when he suffers, since he is anxious to get at the cause of his sufferings, to learn who has produced them and whether it is just or unjust that he should have to bear them. All the results of individuality of separate self-hood involve suffering. It is the surest means of making them truthful to themselves. The suffering of youth is a means of communication, a consequence of hostility, a symbol of threat to the integrity of the body, all calling for help. Suffering does not ennoble, it degrades. It makes adolescents selfish, mean, vindictive, petty, suspicious. It absorbs them in small things; it makes them less than men and women. But in the shaping of inner beliefs, what they are made to suffer and to endure counts more than all we may glean in the unravelling realms of medical science. The parent bears with equanimity the sufferings of youth, but it is the special vocation of the doctor to grow familiar with sufferings and provide the help.

The adolescent is charged with conflicting forces, some exerting pressure towards acceptance of the outer world and others exerting pressure in the opposite direction. Neither of these urges are pleasant for there is no gain without pain. It accompanies reactions involving losses, renunciations, and retaliation. The first waves of suffering following frustration are humility and fear, jealousy and rage, or whatever may lead to retreat or counterattacks. In any case, the pain does not disappear, for new pains are added as readjustments are attempted. Persistence of suffering seems necessary for the pursuit of better solutions to the problems of maturation. Youth learns resignation not from his own suffering but from the suffering of others. The external hope held out for every adolescent sufferer is the confidant and/ or physician. But long before he consults either friend, he does something hazardous on his own to find a more comfortable position. He may resort to drinking, drugs, resolute denial, and bizarre instructions. All of these rarely abate the chronic suffering as a nagging insistence towards finding better solutions. Sometimes youth learns to bear suffering stoically and gets along with it or makes a kind of unpleasant old friend of his misery. The most poignant suffering derives from the loss of satisfaction and opportunity, failure of production and achievement. A sense of unworthiness and uselessness augments as does the painful memory of plan and promise.

The perception of suffering and the capacity to endure it are ever individual. Some develop an acquired indifference to it as one of the secondary symptoms; some suffer little from their sense of guilt, social aggression, or painful maturation; others make a virtue of their vices and pride themselves on their callousness even though suffering is more conducive to effective solutions; still others depend on drugs to bring about temporary serenity. The time may come when drugs will be available to evoke aspiration, spur learning, displace wastefulness, and increase a sense of sans souci. What youth needs is not to care less but to care more, for there is no drug to keep the soul alert with noble discontent. Drugs cannot inspire or encourage or comfort; only a person can heal a person. Chronic suffering and the pervading sense of inadequacy cannot be relieved by drugs. The feeling of inadequacy is accented as a correct self-judgment and an alibi against improvement. The establishment of relationships with fellow human beings is the basic architecture of normal life. If youth is not frozen in his primary narcissism or drowned in secondary narcissism which develops from previous failures, he will strive to find persons about him to have communion. He will keep reaching out first, receiving, and then giving, making acquaintances and then friends, and finding more and more satisfaction in identifications. Socialization is not endless mutual hand-holding but positive relationship, productive and satisfying to lonesome youth.

The adolescent phenomenon in the varying cultures hasn't changed much since the eighth century B.C., but the rapidly altered life-styles and extensive changes in child rearing and in world affairs have made current adolescence a more difficult period for youth, parents and for society. Four categories of adolescents now emerge, two of which are the swinging but stable youth who have the innate power to shape the future. The constructive type is uninvolved and untroubled who takes on some of the external features of his peers but remains oblivious to social unrest and teenage turbulence. Another constructive type is ever-troubled, asks questions and wants quick answers, strives for early assumption of identity and responsibility, participates in debates and protests but expresses deep-seated concern through traditional channels.

A third type, an obstructive, is the hippy in communal quarters away from the parental hearth, withdrawn into a subculture with its own rules and values. He experiments with drugs and resorts to delinquent behavior in protest about mankind but can do nothing about it and wouldn't know how. A fourth type, a destructive, is a street person who adopts violence to destroy the establishment without offering any positive solutions. This lost flower youth of the streets has wilted and love has taken on an angry face, a state of affairs that must not be allowed to continue. The adolescent strivings that make themselves felt over the whole world must be met fortuitously and must be given reality by personal confrontation.

If we face the issue honestly, it is clear that young people live in a world that does not provide them with a reasonable choice for a decent future. The world is changing so rapidly that it is impossible to plan for the future. The values of the past have little meaning—hence the drive to live in the present and get the most out of every moment; that means living with conflict, confrontation, demandingness and violence. Life is intolerable where there is no reverence for the past and little hope for the future. There are always new solutions for youthful problems and each young person must be stimulated to apply them individually and opportunely. We must listen and learn to understand before acting, suspend moralistic judgments, support what seems vital in others, and have the courage to be moved and changed in the process of helping others to move and change.

Design for Living

Youth is not only a reservoir of habits, memories, and attitudes but a designer of a personal life style transforming living data from within and without. This symbol-making function of the mind is one of the primary activities, like eating, looking or moving about. It is his unique interpretation of reality, which may or may not correspond with actual reality that forms his philosophy of living. He is self-reflecting with an ability to objectify himself, consider the kind of being he is, and what he wants to become. It isn't important to come out on top but to come out alive. When we know his design for living we know him. Whatever the social forces, they will somehow accommodate to the human design for youth. He will fulfill the satisfaction of his survival needs by two cerebral forces that keep him alive with food, shelter and sex and keep him loving life itself. He wants security rather than liberty to protect gains made and to advance further, but one cannot learn to swim and keep one foot on the ground. He craves order in his life to guide his actions positively with the prospect of enlarging the range of his satisfactions. The essence of life is to be found in the frustrations of order, the act of progress is to preserve order amid change and preserve change amid order.

Youth is truly a creature of hope, always dissatisfied and never fully adapted to his environment. There is the around-the-corner hope that prompts others and the distant hope that acts as an opiate. Strong hope is a greater stimulant of life than any single realized joy could ever be to lead youth by an agreeable route to make choices in exercising his capacity. He wants independent choice, whatever it may cost and wherever it may lead, even though he often experiences more regret over the past he left than pleasure over the part he preferred. His great difficulty in life is optimal choice. Curiously enough the ponderous nervous system precludes perception from being instantly transformed into reaction. There seems to be an interval for choice, a momentary pause between perception and reaction that stirs imagination to create images and ideas; in fact, the whole mental life of youth is thus built up. He does not immediately react, he does not immediately get what he wants, so he figures the want to himself and creates an image. This constitutes the basis of creativity in solving problems, the outcome, the reflection of youth's unsatisfied desires.

Youth requires freedom to exercise his choices. To the immature youth freedom presents no problem; it means absence of restraint, free to do as he pleases. Such unbridled license leads to social chaos to which all freedom is lost. The freedom that matters is the freedom to know, the freedom of thought, of opinion, of discussion, of action. Youth seeks freedom in fulfillment, to make the utmost of his life by his own efforts, to develop himself as a personage, to give his talents full scope, to live according to ideals, to control his destiny. But freedom involves not only rights but duties. Everything that is really great and inspiring is created by youth who can labor in freedom. To know how to be free is nothing; the arduous thing is to know what to do with freedom. The free way of life proposes ends but it does not prescribe means. Too much freedom too soon becomes an unbearable burden; it always involves learning of responsibility and ability to take advantage of it wisely. The Soviet definition of freedom is "recognition of necessity" limited to those periods of life when they are willing to let others define their needs.

Youth craves personal dignity. It is not in what he does, but in what he understands. It lifts him in mind and heart by the creative union of perception and grace. It is never diminished by the indifference of others. Youth develops personal significance which he shares with others. If this ceases to confirm assumptions or enrich values, his sense of self-constancy becomes insecure, alienated, or he seeks new significance, new loyalties. Youth seeks a sense of worthwhileness, a human value that can be increased in terms of others. He must always decide how he is valuable rather than how valuable he is. It gives him a sense of personal worth and self-respect—the cornerstone of all virtues.

Youth experiences the ultimate concern seeking an explanation of the universe in which he finds himself. He needs a faith, a hope and a purpose to live by and give meaning to his existence through love. He experiences an evolution of love, to love of mankind, to love of God, for love unites without casting off diversity to achieve self-transcendence. He yearns for self-respect and for the respect of others. He is groping in the dark to discover an opening toward new opportunities for living. He becomes self-assertive and may break away from society to the detriment of his maturation. Healthy growth is fostered by love and stunted by egoism. Self-fulfillment is possible only through love for and in a spiritual union with others.

Youth seeks some system of beliefs as safe guides in the midst of uncertainties. It consists of the faith that is in him; he is whatever his faith is. It is an anchoring point, a certainty to serve as a beacon light to assuage him during frustration, anxiety and difficulty. He tends to choose the religion adapted to his spiritual makeup, a religion which may or may not be the formal one in which he was brought up. It constitutes a spiritual gain for future generations in the diverse historic religions of our time. Life with a purpose stands and falls with the religious system. Thoughtful youth with ultimate concern realizes that he is not just a behaving unit because he can look within himself, behold his own conscious individuality, and appreciate the wonder of his unique self-conscious existence, participating in fellowship, beauty, harmony, truth and love in the midst of the mindless universe. Veered toward attainment of material culture, youth will pursue physical pleasure, hobbies, and entertainment; but guided by visionary leaders, he will attain the unification of creativity and happiness in the cause of a transcendental way of life.

Youth wants his aspirations fulfilled in a provident society. A definite moral objective precludes the shearers and the shorn. He demands a return to the personal I-and-thou relationship for exercising his innate abilities. It becomes the framework for a balanced work life with educational, social and political aspects taking precedence over the economic. Society is a kind of parent to youth; if both are to thrive, the values must be clear, coherent and acceptable. The principles of a good society call for a concern with an order of being—which cannot be proved existentially to the sense organs—where it matters greatly that youth be inviolable, that reason shall regulate the will, that truth shall prevail over error. Then will leaders of industry think greatly of their responsibilities to youth for optimal growing, for optimal becoming, for optimal maturing.

REFERENCES

Ansbacher, H. L.: Life style. *J. Individ. Psychol.*, 23:191-212, 1967.

Ashley-Montagu, M. F.: *On Being Human.* London, Abelard-Schuman, 1957.

Berman, S.: Alienation: an essential process of the psychology of adolescence. *J. Am. Acad. Child Psychiatry*, 9:233-250, 1970.

Blos, P.: *On Adolescence.* New York, The Free Press, 1962.

Cantril, B.: *The Human Design.* New York, American Society of Adlerian Psychology, 1964.

Carrighar, S.: *Wild Heritage.* Boston, Houghton Mifflin, 1965.

Cox, R. D.: *Youth into Maturity.* New York, Mental Health Materials Center, 1970.

Dobzhansky, T.: *The Biology of Ultimate Concern.* The New American Library, 1967.

Dowvan, E. *et al.*: *The Adolescent Experience.* New York, John Wiley & Sons, 1966.

Elliott, K. (Ed.): *The Family and its Future*, a Ciba Foundation Symposium. London, J. & A. Churchill, 1970.

Ellison, S. E.: The doctor and the adolescent. *Lancet*, 1:1068, 1971.

Erickson, E. H.: Identity and the life cycle. *Psychol. Issues*, Vol. 1, 1959.

Eslinger, G.: A philosophy of living. *Cerebral Palsy Rev.*, March 1965.

Falkner, F. (Ed.): *Human Development.* Philadelphia, Saunders, 1966.

Frommer, E. A.: *Voyage Through Childhood into the Adult World.* New York, Pergamon, 1969.

Hall, E. T.: *The Hidden Dimension.* Garden City, Doubleday, 1966.

Hill, J. P. *et al.*: *Readings in Adolescent Development.* Englewood Cliffs, Prentice-Hall, 1971.

Joselyn, I. M.: *The Adolescent and his World.* New York, Family Service Association of America, 1957; Adolescents: everyone's special concern. *Int. J. Psychiatry*, 5:478-83, 1968.

Keniston, K.: Youth: A new stage of life. *American Scholar*, 39:631-653, 1970.

Kugelmass, I. N.: *Wisdom with Children.* New York, Day, 1965.

Laufer, M.: *Danger Signs and Prediction in Adolescence*, Case Conference, 1966, Vol. 13.

Lewis, Melvin: *Clinical Aspects of Child Development.* Philadelphia, Lea & Febiger, 1971.

Maier, H. W., *et al.*: *Three Theories of Child Development.* New York, Harper & Row, 1969.

Mays, J. B.: The Adolescent in Modern Society. *Public Health,* Vol. 80, p. 246.

Mead, M.: The Changing Status of Adolescents in the Modern World. *Md. State Med. J.,* p. 61, Nov. 1969.

Medovy, H.: Adolescents: Past, Present and Future. *Can. J. Public Health,* 62:199-204, 1971.

Menninger, R.: What Troubles our Troubled Youth? *Ment. Hyg.,* 52:323-9, 1968.

Milman, D. H.: Adolescence: a Subculture in United States Society. *Bull. N. Y. Acad. Med.,* Vol. 41, No. 4, April 1965.

Newman, E.: The Fruits of Maturity. *J. Am. Geriatr. Soc.,* Vol. 17, No. 9, 1969.

Pearson, G. H. J.: *Adolescence and the Conflict of Generations.* New York, Norton, 1958.

Platt, J. R.: *Man and the Indeterminacies.* New York, John Wiley & Sons, 1966.

Semmens, J. P. *et al.*: *The Adolescent Experience.* New York, Macmillan, 1970.

Whipple, D. V.: *Dynamics of Development.* New York, McGraw-Hill, 1966.

Williams, R. J.: *The Human Frontier.* New York, Harcourt, Brace, 1946.

Winnicott, D. W.: *The Family and Individual Development.* Tavistock Publications, 1965.

Woodmansey, A. C.: The Common Factor in Problems of Adolescence. *Br. J. Med. Psychol.,* 42:353, 1969.

Workman, S. L.: Adolescence: the American predicament. *Clin. Proc. Child. Hosp. D.C.,* 1965.

Young, H. B.: Special Needs of Adolescents. *Int. J. Psychiatry,* 5:494-5, 1968.

CHAPTER II

PHYSICAL IMMATURITY

Man looks about the Universe in awe at its wonders
And forgets that he himself is the greater wonder of all.

Wonderfully and fearfully made. The adolescent form of the growing body completes itself; and the eidos of the personality emerges in the process of becoming. Being is a product; becoming is a process; but the adolescent is in continuous process, i.e. being in becoming. Thales stressed being while Heraclitus stressed becoming. The process of being and becoming is the fusion of two aspects of existence viewed in the light of the current quantum theory applicable to maturation. The developmental tempo of the normal adolescent enables attainment of physical and sexual maturity much earlier than in previous generations, but that of the immature youth proceeds at a slower rate, requiring therapeutic and chemical catalysis to achieve the level of maturation compatible with his heredity and constitution.

The normal adolescent has a vast array of attributes which are measurable and deviated in varying degrees, but the immature youth bears deviations that grow worse with time and interfere with the structural and functional effectiveness of his living transactions. Furthermore, the many changes accompanying adolescence alter some of the body's defense mechanisms against disease which may induce a vicious cycle in suppressing growth and development. Susceptibility to tuberculosis is higher during adolescence but rheumatic fever declines; and thyrotoxicosis, especially in girls, is more common than at any other period in life.

The adolescent sensations of inadequacy are uncontrollable impulses disturbing the equilibrium of body, mind and soul, often appeased by esoteric interests, perfectionism, asceticism, idealism never apparent in the past. The mind must be healed along with the inadequate body. It is in such moments of despair that youth recognizes that he lives not alone but chained to a

40

creature of another world who has no knowledge of him, and by whom it is impossible to make himself understood—his body. What is more important in an adolescent's life than his body? It is like a chemical plant with a thousand windows. We look into one window of the plant when we investigate one aspect of the developmental immaturity. The true mystery of the physique is the visible, not the invisible, but we must probe all.

TABLE I

DEVELOPMENTAL STAGES

(Erikson)

Age	Stage	Maturation		Functions
1	Infancy	Physical		Trust vs. Mistrust
2			Sensory Motor	Autonomy vs. Doubt
3	Preschool	Emotional		Imitative vs. Guilt
4				
5				
6	School	Social		
7				
8				
9			Operational Thinking	Industry vs. Inferiority
10				
11				
12	Puberty	Sexual		
13				
14				
15	Adolescence	Cognitive		
16			Formal Thinking	Identity vs. Diffusion
17				
18				
19	Adulthood	Generative		Intimacy vs. Isolation
20				
21			Hominism	
22	Maturity	Integrative		Integrity vs. Despair
23				
24				

Body Immaturity of Adolescent Boys

The world considers a good exterior a silent recommendation; only in unimportant things does it not trust to appearance, and youth knows it. Any deviation in physical appearance causes adolescent anxiety because it evokes criticism from his peers. The American ideal is youth—handsome, empty youth—expecting the male to be tall with large shoulders, barrel-chest and narrow hips. Besides, boys want to be tall as a symbol of masculinity and as a mark of social advantage; a group always selects a tall boy for the leader. The short, mature boy is better off socially than the short, immature boy, although both feel handicapped. The rate of physical growth suddenly rises from the slow, steady progress in childhood to individual increases determined by physiologic rather than chronological age in adolescence.

Normal variations for the onset of accelerated growth reveal a six-year span, nine to fifteen years in boys and eight to fourteen years in girls. Some become physical adults four years after the first sign of puberty while others require eight years to reach the same physical end-point. Lack of coordination is inevitable with different rates of development in different parts of the body. One youth has years of marked embarrassment, terrified about the possible permanence of his small stature, while another feels that he will never stop growing. There is short-waistedness due to the growth of legs disproportionate to the trunk, increase in hip width before shoulder width, growth of one part of the face before another, and increase in muscle massiveness before muscle strength. The rates of genital and sex-linked anatomic changes exceed the rate of change in other organs. Physical disability thus becomes augmented at the expense of physical appearance. A boy remains about two years behind a girl of the same age throughout adolescence.

Youth expects every morning to open into a new world for him, finds that today is like yesterday, and still believes tomorrow will be different. He has no fear of facing life. He champs at the bit. The jealousies, the trials, the sorrows of life of man do not intimidate the young. Youth needs no ideal; it has one already, which is youth itself and the wondrous diversity of life—private life—the only real one full of passion. Not so with the immature boy who expects equality and finds frustrations, who seeks happiness and finds only misery; yet growth is invested with symbolic meaning so that physical maturation implies growth in other areas as well. Conformance for peer acceptance is the great goal with a sex-appropriate appearance. Psychological changes accompany physical variation in appearance, for exaggeration of individual differences in physique creates considerable self-consciousness.

A boy's adolescent growth spurt begins with increase in the size of the genitals, followed by appearance of ancillary hair, beginning of a beard, deepening of the voice, increase in muscular strength, and development of other secondary sex characteristics. Eventually, he develops broader shoulders, narrow hips, long arms, especially forearms and legs. Sex-type differences extend to more subtle distinctions in movement, hairiness, skin texture, asymmetry of features, and body language to influence the boy's thinking of himself and his treatment of others. Sex-inappropriate physique occurs early in puberty with slow physical development. The boy tends to deposit a fat girdle around the hips and thighs accompanied by small primary sex characteristics and subcutaneous tissue about the nipples. There may be gynecomastia with slight temporary enlargement of nodules and tenderness about the nipples after genital growth has started, but before other secondary sex characteristics have become pronounced. Boys worry about sex inappropriateness of facial characteristics, especially unmasculine qualities such as eyeglasses, turned-up nose, dimples, receding chin, small rosebud mouth, lack of beard, protruding ears, alopecia, tooth defects and acne.

Certain adolescent traits have been socially specialized as the appropriate attitudes and behavior of only one sex, while other human traits have been designated for the opposite sex. The social specialization is rationalized into a sound theory that the socially decreed behavior is natural for one sex and unnatural for the other and that the deviant has a developmental or endocrine defect. Inappropriate sex development may thus characterize a boy as girlish because of a slow change of voice, late maturity or a female pattern of fat deposition, though transient. More serious are the problems arising from the supposed lack of sex appropriateness in the maturing male, such as poor stance, lack of muscular strength, sparse beard and physical frailness. Adolescent ideals of sex-appropriate appearance are quite unrealistic; sexual growth is particularly vulnerable to the narrow notions of normality maintained by youth.

The late maturer with developmental lag behind his peers is concerned about his future development. Life becomes one long painful postponement while the future enters into him gradually to transform itself long before it happens. But his preoccupation with the future prevents him from seeing the present as it is and prompts him to rearrange the past unless steps are taken to shape his developmental future. Such a boy competes well with his peers for a while until he begins to withdraw from group activities. After school, he gravitates towards the younger boys closer to his own physical developmental level. But he can achieve high stations in recreational or institutional groups with boy scouts or church groups. Immaturity in one area of development often contradicts normal or superior maturation in other areas. The late maturer is more introspective, sensitive, insightful in dealing with the problem of others because of his own experience in coping with delayed maturation. How shall one so weak in adolescence become strong in adulthood? He only changes his fancies if the doctor induces optimal maturation.

Body Immaturity of Adolescent Girls

Adolescent girls like excess of any quality. Without knowing, they want to suffer, and to suffer they must exaggerate. And so they become introspective to get at the cause of suffering, to find the way out, and whether it is just or unjust that they should have to bear it. Nothing induces more suffering than physical inadequacy. Pain makes them think, thought makes them wise, and wisdom makes life endurable. And the lot of young men and women is equally painful in the realm of immaturity. The roles of today's men and women tend to merge with males less masculine and females less feminine. They feel less need to conform and so it is difficult to tell boys from girls and girls from boys. Such freedom creates confusion; confusion, anxiety; and anxiety, unrest. Nevertheless, there comes a time in adolescence when all girls want to become womanly.

Variations in physical appearance and rate of maturation cause such anxiety in the adolescent girl because she feels different from her peers. The physician must reassure the girl of the temporary nature of these variations while correcting deviations from the desired pattern. But it is often difficult for the male physician to empathize with the female adolescent. There is nothing so difficult to support imperturbably as the head of a lovely girl, except her grief. Appearance is uppermost in her mind but shyness precludes mention of deviations. A fixed anxiety about appearance is less disturbing than a floating anxiety about her life. Much anxiety stems from the importance a girl places on the critical attitudes of others about her appearance, for near to her heart is her own beauty or charm. She is more concerned about her physical development than the adolescent boy because outer appearance and inner self are more closely bound in the female. It is easy to be beautiful but difficult to appear so. Youth is right, for only shallow people do not judge by appearance.

The adolescent girl rarely complains about shortness unless it is combined with obesity. Tallness disturbs her; she stoops because of the self-conscious effort to compensate for height and breast development. Tallness hinders a girl in social relationships with boys because boys tend to be shorter in early adolescence and the reverse is the cultural ideal. Sex-inappropriate characteristics to an adolescent girl include tallness, squattiness, large hands and feet, clumsy ankles, large breasts, pigmented facial hair, extreme thinness, obesity, heavy lower jaw, hairy arms and legs and massive body build. Unfeminine facial features include glasses, braces, large nose, massive mouth, receding chin, acne, moles, birthmarks, scars, large pores, oily skin and freckles.

LACK OF ADEQUATE WEIGHT FOR BODY BUILD

The adolescent is weighed in the balances and found wanting. Body weight and body build are primarily determined by genetic factors; the offspring resembles his parent. Sex, dietary habits and exercise determine chemical composition in terms of lean tissue and fat. The male body contains more lean muscular tissue; the female, a higher percentage of body fat; but in either, eating more than necessary increases body fat, and active exercise increases musculature. Appreciable gain in weight in days is due to rapid increase in body water, for synthesis of new protoplasm proceeds very slowly in weeks at a rate of 150 gms/day. Accumulation of neutral fat occurs rapidly on high caloric diets in the underweight individual.

Weight is the simplest criterion of body composition, a function of body size. In low weight for body build, the intravascular phase shows a loss of red cell mass with an increase in plasma volume, resulting in a drop in total blood volume. Body water and intracellular phase are like plasma volume, relatively high for the new weight. By contrast, the intercellular phase and certain body solids and fat are very low. Weight loss due to tissue dissolution occurs much more rapidly than weight gain. Fat oxidation rates are markedly accelerated and tissue loss may be as rapid as 500 gms/day and water loss from the digestive tract about ten times as fast—5000 gms/day. Short-time rapid weight loss signifies either desalting water loss or true dehydration, whichever fits the circumstances. Weight loss and undernutrition result from negative nutrient balance with consequent impairment of body structure, function and maturation in a variety of systemic disorders.

TABLE II

WEIGHT AND HEIGHT MEASUREMENTS OF ADOLESCENTS
(Percentiles)

		3		50		97	
		Male	Female	Male	Female	Male	Female
10 Years							
	Weight, pounds	56.7	53.2	72	70.2	100	102
	Height, inches	50.7	50.2	55.2	54.5	59.2	58.7
12 Years							
	Weight, pounds	67.2	63.5	84.5	87.5	124.2	127.7
	Height, inches	54.5	55.2	59	59.7	63.7	64.7
14 Years							
	Weight, pounds	79.7	83	107.5	108.5	150.5	150.7
	Height, inches	57.5	58.2	64	62.7	69.7	67.2
16 Years							
	Weight, pounds	103.5	91.7	129.7	117	170.5	157.7
	Height, inches	61.5	59.5	67.7	64	73	67.7
18 Years							
	Weight, pounds	113	94.5	139	120	179	160.7
	Height, inches	62.7	59.5	68.7	64	74	67.7

Weight-loss Syndromes

Nutritional deficiencies induce loss of weight from interference with ingestion, absorption, storage, or utilization of food or from increased excretion, excess loss in congenital defects, from chromosomal anomalies and inborn errors of metabolism and from hematologic, vascular, parasitic, collagen and neoplastic diseases.

Anorexia nervosa causes progressive weight loss with emaciation from strange diets, aversion to all food, and eating at times to relieve anxiety, especially in girls. There may be a craze for slimming, a desire to excite sympathy or to attract attention. It is a disturbance in the body image and perception of the bodily state with a paralyzing ineffectiveness. She may deny being thin or tired or infantile. She is a perfectionistic, obsessive, compulsive with food as an obsessive thought and avoidance of food a compulsive act. The symptoms represent an attempt to escape from adult sexual roles in the service of regaining control of the body, the self and the parents. The neurotic heredofamilial syndrome has a mortality rate up to 15 percent and a morbidity rate of 35 percent from chronic pathology and/or sexual dysfunction.

Hyperthyroidism develops during puberty in irritable unstable girls. There is loss of weight, lassitude and fatigue despite adequate food intake, causing home conflicts, school difficulties and poor grades. A familial tendency to thyroid disease and genetic mode of inheritance combine with the long-acting stimulator LATS in the 7S Y-globulin fraction to produce hyperthyroidism. The thyroid gland is insensitive to a reduction of pituitary thyrotropic secretion, or the hypothalamus-pituitary axis is insensitive to increased blood levels or to thyroid hormone. The diagnosis is determined from exophthalmos, large goiter, signs of hypermetabolism, ^{131}I uptake at four and twenty-four hours.

Simmonds' disease is marked cachexia due to progressive insufficiency of the adenohypophysis. It may commence at puberty with marked loss of weight, lowered BMR, thinning of sexual hair, atrophy of the breasts in females, atrophic changes in the genitalia, loss of libido in the male and amenorrhea in the female, and sterility in both sexes with diminished urinary excretion of 17-ketosteroids, 17-hydroxycorticoids and FSH.

Tuberculosis is a chance infection from an active focus. It is a worldwide problem of a single disease entity with the portal of entry in the adolescent lungs that creates complications in any part of the body. There is unexplained fever, persistent fatigue, loss of weight, failure to thrive, with or without signs of pneumonia. The tuberculous endothoracic lesion may be of the classic primary type; it may be of the chronic reinfection type; or it may be mixed. Prognosis is good in the light of improved diagnostic techniques and clinical therapeutic agents.

Diabetes mellitus presents keto-acidosis as the first manifestation and weight loss in significant amount. However, cachexia may develop slowly during the development of diabetes or may become marked in a diabetic poorly controlled with diet and insulin. An adolescent with progressive weight loss should have the urine examined for glucose, especially with a familial incidence of diabetes, recurrent skin infections, subtle changes in thirst and frequent urination. The diabetic state may become manifest after recovery from infections with an inability to regain weight, and the development of progressive fatigue, polyuria and thirst.

Addison's disease develops insidiously with anorexia, loss of weight, lassitude and digestive disorder. The craving for salt may not be apparent, hyperpigmentation of the skin not discernible, laboratory procedures misleading. Serum electrolyte levels are affected by dehydation but hyperkalemia is always a reliable finding. Urinary and plasma corticoids and response to ACTH are critical procedures for estimating adrenocortical insufficiency. Normal levels of urinary 17-OCHS do not rule out the presence of Addison's disease. A summer hazard is excessive loss of salt and water associated with anorexia, fever, dehydration, nausea, vomiting and abdominal pain, hence activity should be restricted during hot and humid weather, and salt and sweetened fluids should be increased.

Treatment of malnutrition, reflected by loss of weight, decreased muscle mass and lowered serum protein levels, involves correction of protein-caloric deficiency. The clinical spectrum ranges in a variety of forms characterized by growth retardation, on the one hand, to marked marasmus, on the other. Weight loss is accompanied by fatigue, lassitude, restlessness, and irritability, as well as anorexia, digestive disorders and constipation. There is a limited attention span and increased susceptibility to infection. Muscular development is inadequate, muscles are flabby, posture fatigued, shoulders rounded, chest flat, complexion muddy, eyes dull. The undernourished body is characterized by too little fat; too little lean tissue; too much water, too much of which is extracellular; a large plasma volume; a small erythrocyte volume, yielding a low hematocrit in relatively high blood volume with hyponatremia and bodily hypotonicity, hypoproteinemia, and slight hyperkalemia.

An adolescent diet, quantitatively and qualitatively inadequate, may be due to low food production, inadequate preservation, restricted purchasing power, poor food habits and deficient knowledge of the relation between diet and health. Excessive incidence of infectious disease may be due to poor environmental conditions, poor personal hygiene and insufficient health services. Nutritional therapy must be individualized. An adequate and balanced diet should be formulated, supplemented by vitamin concentrates. Where anorexia prevails, food should be given in concentrated form but the fat content kept low. Snacks between meals are permitted if they do not interfere with appetite for the next meal. Quiet periods of fifteen minutes before meals may abolish tension. Outdoor activity should be encouraged for sedentary youths and group play for the loners.

LACK OF ADEQUATE HEIGHT FOR BODY BUILD

Growth is the only evidence of life. Longitudinal growth is achieved by the interposition of a soft structure to allow interstitial growth. These growth plates provide the right balance between sufficient softness to allow interstitial growth and sufficient hardness to form part of the skeleton. Any abnormality may upset the balance that leads to growth failure. Some creatures grow throughout life, but man grows only unto maturity for the growth plate has built-in obsolescence. Not only does the growth plate stop producing bone, but it disappears almost completely, consumed by its own product. During adolescence most growth discs are closed by adrenal androgens, but growth cartilage underlying articular cartilage remains dormant throughout life.

Chemically, growth is the replication of DNA and accretion of protein. The former eventuates because genes, functional demands or release hormones that promote growth or modify structure, and the new DNA so formed, have jurisdiction over a new volume of cytoplasm. Growth retardation, therefore, is failure of cell multiplication, failure of DNA synthesis, or of protein synthesis. Thus, it is to be expected that under abnormal conditions, hormones no longer exert their optimal effects and dietary intake would not increase with time and age. Wasting of energy or of protein may occur due to some abnormal situation which might enhance growth mechanisms temporarily, but the losses of energy and protein may be too great for physiologic adjustment to compensate.

TABLE III

MEASURE OF OSSEOUS DEVELOPMENT
(Comparison of chronologic and bone ages)

Age

10 years   Wrist-pisiform.

12 years   External condyle of humerus.
Union of trochlea and capitellum of humerus.

14 years   Union of proximal epiphysis of radius.
Union of olecranon and ulna.

16 years   Union of epiphyses of metacarpals and metatarsals.
Appearance of crest of ilium.

18 years   Union of distal epiphysis of radius and of ulna.
Union of distal epiphysis of tibia and of fibula.

Short Stature in Adolescents

Height is the best guide of overall growth-plate activity. Shortness below the third percentile for height may be the presenting symptom of many disorders due to alteration in the speed of growth of an otherwise normal plate or to sluggishness of a growth plate hampered by abnormal architecture. Stature must be assessed in relation to chronological age or to bone age. If a boy is tall for his chronological age, he will become a tall man if the bone age corresponds, but if the bone age is ahead of the chronological age, he will mature more quickly and his final height will be below normal. Linear growth and skeletal maturity are normally interrelated but become dissociated by growth-plate disease. Local growth is affected by architectural disorders of the growth plate but bone age is hormonally determined.

Growth in height is a direct function of skeletal height determined by the growth of the long bones of the legs. The adolescent height cycle starts abruptly with rapid acceleration in the rate of growth, increases progressively for a year, and reaches the maximal increment in mid-adolescence. This is followed by a progressive reduction of growth during late adolescence until the growth rate reaches the level normal for earlier childhood. But the rate of growth gradually tapers further so that all growth ceases in boys at seventeen three-fourth years ± ten months, and in girls at sixteen one-half years ± thirteen months. Shortness in adolescent boys induces both physical and emotional immaturity.

Growth fulfillment according to genetic potential is the most sensitive index of an adolescent's health status. Heredity sets growth limits; environment determines the exact position within these limits. Shortness of stature combined with deficit in weight indicates longstanding undernutrition or disease that produces endocrine as well as GH deficiency. The size of the siblings, parents and other blood relatives as well as individual variants in the growth pattern must be taken into consideration in the evaluation. Some children grow slowly for several years but eventually attain their genetic potential. They lag behind their peers, but their height and sexual maturation ages correspond with their radiologic bone ages. However, delayed adolescence with a retarded growth spurt is compensated by prolonged duration of growth.

A satisfactory adolescent height means that low weight reflects somatic or recent illness. If height and weight are both proportionately reduced, the adolescent will have a deceptively healthy appearance. The underlying basis may be genetic or indicate ill-health or undernutrition. If the body proportions are abnormal for age and particularly if the extremities are short, the underlying cause is in the skeletal system. Poor growth is usually due to inadequate food intake. The diagnostic value of the response to an adequate diet under controlled conditions must not be overlooked in avoiding unnecessary examinations.

The rate of growth in height is affected by the genetic, nutritional and endocrine status, accelerated by gonadal steroids and thyroid hormones. A growth problem may involve a deficiency of the growth hormone which stimulates the rate of growth but not the rate of skeletal maturation, and a deficiency of androgen which accelerates both rate of growth and rate of skeletal maturation. Cortisol and its analogues inhibit growth in pharmacologic doses and slow the rate of skeletal maturation. Thyroid hormone is essential for a complete response to the growth hormone rather than merely a stimulator, because its absence retards the rate of growth and skeletal maturation. Inadequate supply of thyroid hormone diminishes the secretion of the growth hormone. The short stature of a child with skeletal dystrophy will not respond to growth-producing stimuli, for diminution of growth is limited by androgen and estrogen with premature fusion of the epiphyses. Any interference with the rate of production of the growth hormone by the anterior pituitary will affect growth. CNS and hypothalamus regulate pituitary activity, yet nutritional deficiency remains a determining factor in the development of a short child.

Hormonal deficiency may be genetically determined, hence endocrine and genetic factors both may determine short stature. Even if the growth disturbance is hormonal in origin, the cause is not primarily a growth hormone disturbance. Normal growth requires optimal thyroxin, hydrocortisone and insulin in addition to growth hormone. At puberty, the normal pubertal growth spurt can occur only if the proper gonadal hormone, testosterone or estradiol, is present. For example, deficient thyroxin causes short stature because the bones do not increase in length fast enough. Still, growth hormone plays a role because hypothyroidism both diminishes growth hormone secretion and impedes the action of GH secreted. Excessive hydrocortisone stunts growth by inhibiting GH secretion.

Androgen deficiency in a puberal male halts the puberal growth spurt and so the bony epiphyses remain unfused. Slow growth of the long bones continues longer than usual and final height may be increased. Excessive androgen causes an initial growth spurt but fuses the bony epiphyses before normal puberty and stunts growth. Once again, the growth spurt induced by testosterone at puberty may be due to GH rather than to testosterone, since patients with normal but delayed puberty have a mild GH secretion deficiency which can be corrected by testosterone administration.

TABLE IV

LABORATORY TESTS FOR SHORT STATURE

Urine: Color and odor, organic acids, mucopolysaccharides, reducing substances, amino acids, amino acid chromatography.

Blood: Hemogram, blood cell anomalies, iron deficiency, fasting glucose, BUN, protein, Na, K, Cl, CO_2, pH, Ca, P, alkaline phosphate, uric acid, cholesterol, immunoelectrophoresis.

Special Tests: Nuclear sex for all females, karyotype for multiple anomalies, EEG for seizures, sweat test for fibrocystic disease, stool ova and parasites, protein-losing enteropathy, saccharide anomalies.

X-ray Films: Chest, skull, hemiskeleton for bone age, intravenous pyelogram.

Hormone Assays: True thyroxine, ^{131}I, urinary 17-KS and 17-OHCS, metyrapone test, growth hormone assay.

Diagnosis of the underlying cause requires systematic investigations. Fifty syndromes are characterized by short stature; some are low birth-weight dwarfs with growth failure before birth and birth weight below that expected for the period of gestation; some require no more than the knowing-eye of the experienced clinician; some can be detected with a computer; some can be delineated by careful examination and/or a few selected tests; and some preclude delineation despite investigation. Decision must therefore be made whether the child is normal with short stature or has hypopituitarism, or belongs to an unexplained group of dwarfism.

Mild hypothyroidism may be difficult to detect but must be considered in any child with growth failure. Excessive corticosteroid retards growth more than Cushing's syndrome. Chromosome disorders such as gonadal dysgenesis are frequent causes, hence buccal smears should be made to determine sex chromosomes. However, when gonadal dysgenesis is associated with chromosome mosaic, i.e. cell differentiation complements of chromosomes, the buccal smears may be normal and the diagnosis can be made only by further study of the chromosomes. There are some conditions for which treatment is readily available, i.e. malnutrition, anorexia due to emotional deprivation, malabsorption, congenital heart disease or chronic renal disorder. When hypopituitarism is due to a demonstrable CNS lesion, the diagnosis is clear-cut but in the idiopathic type, it is difficult and usually delayed until pituitary failure becomes manifest at the expected age with failure of sex hormone secretion. Availability of human growth hormone makes earlier diagnosis possible by the simple expedient of the therapeutic test.

There is no single reliable diagnostic test for growth hormone deficiency; a battery of tests is required, and even then the underlying cause may not be discernible. Spontaneous hypoglycemia may be a symptom of hypopituitarism. The two most useful tests for detecting hormone deficiency are the plasma growth response to insulin-induced hypoglycemia and the nitrogen retention test during treatment with human growth hormone. A normal response is not diagnostic. The final proof of growth hormone deficiency comes from a significant growth spurt in response to treatment with the hormone. The child whose short stature is not due to GH deficiency obviously does not respond in growth rate although he may develop antibodies to the human hormone that block its effect during the early months of treatment.

Blood counts, urinalysis and tuberculin tests rule out common disorders. Blood urea nitrogen, serum electrolyte and blood pH reveal possible renal disorders. Total serum determinations reflect malnutrition. Serum calcium and inorganic phosphate levels reveal parathyroid disease and hypercalcemia. Glucose tolerance tests suggest pituitary disorders, diabetes mellitus, glycogen storage disease or celiac syndrome. Radiologic bone age enables assessment of the prognosis for makeup growth. A bone age in accord with or in advance of the chronological age points to a negative prognosis, while retarded bone age implies a better potential for growth. Intravenous pyelography unravels renal disorders which may not have produced biochemical lesions. Roentgenograms of the chest diagnose pulmonary tuberculosis, cystic fibrosis of the pancreas, and congenital heart disease. ECG reveals cardiac malformation. Chromosomal tests, urinary examinations for amino-aciduria and tests of endocrine functions are final diagnostic steps. Growth hormone is determined serially by radioimmune assays while Arginine-insulin stimulation for growth is a sequential hospital procedure.

Treatment must be planned to alleviate any underlying disorder. The youth not amenable to treatment must be taught to accept his status and compensate shortness in other ways. After all, many leading figures in sports are short. The drive from within in short stature is unparalleled by any other stimulus for great achievement. Whatever the cause, a decisive corrective measure constitutes optimal nutrition. Linear growth is achieved with human growth hormone when the epiphyses are open. There is retention of N, P, K, Ca and Mg, increased body weight with adequate calories, increased free fatty-acid and blood ketone levels. Glucose tolerance develops with high hormone dosage and may persist long after other changes have returned to base line levels. Growth hormone levels in the blood measured by radio-immuno-assay are about 10 mg/ml/serum. The end-result is accelerated growth with continued response unless HGH binding substances and HGH antibodies appear in the plasma. The only disturbing HGH side-effect is decreased glucose tolerance.

Target gland deficiencies must be corrected since potent growth hormone is not generally available. In thyroid deficiency, thyroid administration up to 100 mg daily may be necessary. In adrenal function deficiency, oral cortisone administration suffices, but high dosage of HGH suppresses growth due to catabolic action. Replacement of sex hormones at the time of expected puberty is particularly effective; a synergistic effect may be produced by combining thyroid with male hormone therapy. Fluoxymesterone 2 mg daily has less effect on bone maturation than methyltestosterone. In girls, it is important to determine whether height or sexual maturity is more desirable. As a rule, growth is stimulated with thyroid and fluoxymesterone until bone age is mature. Virilizing effects such as enlarged clitoris, hair growth and deepening voice must be detected early to reduce the dosage. Later, Premarin® 1.25 mg daily will induce development of secondary sexual characteristics and periodic withdrawal bleeding. Estrogen administration early in the course of treatment has a more specific effect than androgen in causing epiphyseal closure, hence treatment should be delayed until maximum height has been achieved.

Androgen therapy in males produces a growth spurt if the epiphyses are open. There will be broadening of the frame, muscular development, deepening of the voice, increase in penis and prostate size, pubic hair growth within two months accompanied by spontaneous penile erection and nocturnal emissions. Growth rate is maximum in the first year, but the tallest result is about 5 feet 2½ inches. The degree of virilization is below that expected for a similarly treated eunuch. There is interest in the opposite sex but little social adjustment. In females, linear growth occurs on androgen therapy with feminization developing after a change to estrogen. There is breast and nipple development, labial and vaginal maturation and uterine growth. When the estrogen dosage is cycled, menstrual-like vaginal bleeding occurs during withdrawal. Fertility is unlikely yet feminine social adjustment is better than in males as is enjoyment of normal marital status.

TABLE V

UNION OF EPIPHYSES

Boys	Girls	
12 years	12 years	Trochlea and capitellum of humerus.
14 years	13-14 years	Olecranon and ulna.
14 years	13-14 years	Epiphysis of calcaneus.
15-17 years	14-16 years	Proximal epiphysis of radius
15-17 years	14-16 years	Trochanter and head of femur.
16-18 years	15-17 years	Epiphyses of metacarpals and metatarsals.
17 years	18 years	Coracoid.
18-20 years	17-19 years	Distal epiphysis of radius.
18-20 years	17-19 years	Distal epiphysis of ulna.
18-20 years	17-19 years	Distal epiphyses of tibia and fibula.
18-20 years	17-19 years	Acromion.
18-20 years	17-19 years	Head and greater tuberosity to the humerus.
18-20 years	17-19 years	Distal epiphysis of femur.
18-20 years	17-19 years	Proximal epiphyses of tibia and fibula.

Dwarfing Syndromes

Diseases of an organ system may lead to conspicuous growth failure which mimics endocrine disorders, although primary endocrine disease is rarely the cause of growth failure. Short growth becomes evident long before the age of five years in premordial dwarfism, progeria, skeletal dystrophy, congenital hypothyroidism, malabsorption syndrome, and other metabolic disorders. Congenital heart disease interferes with growth in shunts or cyanosis and persists after surgical treatment. Pulmonary disease, especially intractable asthma, leads to short stature, even without steroid therapy. Bronchiectasis, cystic fibrosis, chronic infections and chronic anemia all depress height.

Gastrointestinal disease, especially regional enteritis and cirrhosis of the liver, retards growth though it is not associated with malabsorption. Chronic renal disease depresses the growth rate while chronic infection impairs the functional efficiency of other systems of the body and thus retards growth. Skeletal dystrophy and storage disease impair growth while pseudohypoparathyroidism produces short stature and skeletal malformations. Gonadal dysgenesis is associated with short stature and mental retardation while CNS abnormalities lead to mental and growth retardation. Congenital hypothyroidism slows growth while juvenile hypothyroidism may reveal retarded growth as its only manifestation. Cortical excess due to tumor retards maturation.

Constitutional growth retardation in slow developers appears without congenital defect, neurological disorder, or endocrine stigmata. There is a proportionate growth retardation throughout childhood with the initial height between the third and tenth percentile and the growth pattern following a sequential curve below the tenth percentile. The bone age is below the chronological age and roughly equivalent to the height age. These slow developers do not show the typical adolescent growth spurt and remain the shortest in their group. Pituitary function tests may yield the underlying basis for the familial growth retardation. Emotional deprivation may produce significant retardation in height and skeletal maturation resembling that seen in hypopituitarism. The child emerges at adolescence with emotional instability, mental retardation and motor incoordination. There may be bizarre behavior patterns and specific defects from involvement of the cerebral-hypothalamus-pituitary axis. The endocrine basis for growth retardation is evidenced in the abnormal response to metyrapone and inadequate serum HGH response to hypoglycemia, even though some who are not growing have a normal HGH response.

Congenital hypothyroidism may be due to thyroid dysgenesis or defective hormonal dysgenesis from inborn enzymatic defect, iodine deficiency or maternal ingestion of antithyroid drugs. Early adequate and consistent thyroid therapy produces normal physical growth and development, but late onset of cretinism involves a delay in attaining adult height if epiphyseal fusion occurs. The longer the delay in treatment, the more irreparable the damage of the lack of thyroid on the sensitive brain. Idiopathic hypothyroidism presents a variable onset difficult to assess, for it takes years to develop without thyroid enlargement. Growth failure is the striking clue accompanied by lassitude, pallor, sensitivity to cold, capricious appetite, recurrent infections, persistent anemia and poor schooling.

Hypopituitary disorders involve organic hypopituitarism from isolated deficiencies or combinations of defect of ACTH, TSH, STH, or HGH, and the gonadotropins FSH and LH, and idiopathic hypopituitarism from no detectable organic lesion of the pituitary. Early morning fatigue and hypoglycemia and convulsions in a short adolescent suggests hypopituitarism from ACTH and STH deficiency. The sella turcica may be small and bone age less than the chronological age. Treatment with HGH may be blocked by development of injected HGH antibodies. Thyroid is added in the presence of associated hypothyroidism.

Pseudohypoparathyroidism reveals adequate production of parathyroid hormone but failure of end-organ response to the hormone. It is characterized by a familial incidence with short stature, stocky build, round face, short metacarpal and metatarsal bones. There is mental retardation, calcinosis of the basal ganglia, blue sclerae, defective dentition and osteoporosis.

Diabetes mellitus shifts the bone age in uncontrolled adolescents to the left of the median curve. The mean adult height attained by the juvenile diabetic is less than average for both sexes. Youth unconsciously makes use of his chronic condition to express anxiety about problems involving control of the body and its impulses, and independence from parental restraints. There may be Mauriae syndrome with dwarfism, hepatomegaly and obesity in juvenile diabetes. The long-term outlook for the diabetic adolescent is poor, but it is imperative to control the disease as accurately as possible.

Diabetes insipidus arises from a deficiency of secretions or acceleration of hormone degradation or lack of end-organ response to normal amounts of hormone. The onset of thirst and/or enuresis requires study of accompanying fatigue, irritability, poor growth, weight loss and disturbed sleep. Some may control the disease by drinking enough water not to require exogenous vasopressin; others may require excessive drinking and urination, interfering with all activities. Vasopressin is injected daily, 0.2 ml, gradually increasing the dose to effect a satisfactory balance of water intake and output.

Growth hormone deficiency produces an immature but symmetrical youth. Bony development is slowed in relation to chronological age but equal to the height age. Some growth hormone levels will distinguish the normal from the abnormal. Normal controls respond to insulin-induced hypoglycemia and to arginine infusion with increase in plasma growth hormone. But normal adolescents may exhibit discrepancies in their growth hormone response to these two stimuli, hence both tests are mandatory for absolute diagnosis. Pituitary deficiency may be established by thyroid function tests, TSH, Metropirene stimulation tests, ACTH and twenty-four-hour urine for gonadotropins.

Premordial dwarfism produces the classic dwarf, symmetrical but very small. Bony development coincides with chronological age. Height is significantly decreased, hence epiphyseal closure can be expected at the usual age causing very short stature.

Achondroplasia reveals disproportionately small limbs and a relatively large head. There is protrusion of the abdomen and gluteal region with marked lumbar lordosis and thoracic kyphosis, due to an abnormal endochondro-ossification because of the inability of the epiphyseal plate to produce a sufficient amount of columnal cartilage to produce longitudinal growth of the bone. The gait is waddling, musculature fair, mentality normal.

Chronic lymphocytic thyroiditis develops at puberty, especially in girls. It may show up as asymptomatic goiter with no history of infection or pain in the thyroid region. The gland may be painless though enlarged. The only clue may be the palpable delphian node above the isthmus. The adolescent should be checked for anti-immune bodies, elevated ^{131}I uptake, and failure of TSH to raise ^{131}I uptake.

Macrogenitosomia praecox produces short stature in adolescents subjected to excessive secretion of sex steroids. It increases the skeletal maturation far beyond the chronological age but causes premature fusion of the growth centers.

Gonadal dysgenesis in an adolescent girl with short stature of unknown cause should be tested for the defect regardless of the absence of characteristic facies or anomalies. In half, the cause of the chromosome pattern is mosaic with varying degrees of expression. Turner's syndrome creates multiple anomalies, i.e. short stature, webbed neck, cubitus chest, low hair line, and gonadal aplasia. A short female should have a buccal smear for sex chromatin to demonstrate the usual X-O chromosomal pattern. Elevated gonadotropic levels are secondary to the gonadal defect. Estrogen treatment improves growth but slightly.

Cushing's syndrome causes short stature and obesity from adrenal disease or exogenous medication, the correction of which leads to growth improvement as long as the epiphyses remain open. Precocious development from congenital adrenal hyperplasia and virilizing tumors is characterized by rapid growth in childhood, but early epiphyseal closure leads to short stature. Once the bone age has exceeded the height age, little improvement can be expected in eventual stature.

TABLE VI

SHORT STATURE DISORDERS

Genetic: Intrauterine growth retardation, prematurity, bird-headed dwarfs, leprechaunism, progeria, maternal deprivation, diffuse malignancies, idiopathic hypercalcemia, pseudohypoparathyroidism.

Cardiac: Congenital heart disease, especially cyanotic type.

CNS: Tumors, toxoplasmosis, Riley-Day syndrome, brain defect.

Chromosomal: Chromosomal abnormalities except Klinefelter's (XXY) and metafemale (XXX).

Endocrine: Thyroid deficiency, hypopituitarism, adrenal disorders.

Inborn Errors: Glycogen storage cystinosis, vitamin D refractory rickets, Faconi syndrome, oxalosis, galactosemia, mono- and disaccharide intolerance, defective amino acid synthesis.

Nutritional: Fibrocytic disease, celiac, ulcerative colitis, regional ileitis, hepatic insufficiency, low caloric intake, chronic infection, vitamin A intoxication.

Pulmonary: Chronic lung disease, with functional impairment.

Renal: Metabolic acidosis disorders.

Skeletal: Achondroplasia, chondroectodermal dysplasia, osteogenesis imperfecta, diseases of the epiphysis, diseases of the spine.

PHYSICAL MATURATION

Man is a born child; his power is the power of growth. He takes the longest to mature and is the most helpless during his immaturity. Growth covers a wide variety of diverse complex phenomena involving a series of changes rather than just addition of material to increase size. There are differentiations in all parts of the body to perform discrete functions, as well as alterations in the form of the body as a whole and in its organs and systems. There are additions of material, such as bone; substitutions of material, such as the thymus gland. There are transformations, such as cartilage conversion into bone, and modifications, such as secondary sex changes, in the shape of bony skeleton. Every part of the body grows at its own rate for its own period; the growth of one part being controlled by the activity of another, yielding continuous changes in the body. Yet growth does not cease with maturity since skin, nails, hair, intestinal lining continue to grow throughout life, and nearly every tissue and organ reveal recurring cycles of growth, elimination, and replacement.

Physical Maturation Tests and Measurements

Acheson, R. M.: The Oxford method of assessing skeletal maturity. *Clin. Orthop., 10:*19-39, 1954.

Bayley, N.: Size and body build of adolescents in relation to rate of skeletal maturing. *Child Develop., 14:*47-90, 1943.

————. Tables for predicting adult height from skeletal age and present height. *J. Pediatr., 28:*49-64, 1946.

Falkner, F.: *Human Development.* Philadelphia, Saunders, 1966.

————. The somatic investigations. *Mod. Probl. Pediatr., 5:*70-86, 1960.

Frankenburg, W. K. *et al.*: The Denver developmental screening test. *J. Pediatr., 71:*181, 1967.

Garn, S. M. *et al.*: A rational approach to the assessment of skeletal maturation. *Ann. Radiol. (Paris), 7:*297-307, 1964.

Hayden, F. J.: *Physical Fitness for the Mentally Retarded.* A Manual for Teachers and Parents. Ontario, Metropolitan Toronto Assoc. for Retarded Children, 1964.

Hewitt, D. *et al.*: Some aspects of skeletal development through adolescence. *Am. J. Phys. Anthropol., 19:*321-331, 1961.

Krogman, W. M.: *A Handbook of the Measurement and Interpretation of Height and Weight in the Growing Child.* Monog. of the Soc. for Research in Child Develop., 1948.

Meiks, L. T. *et al.*: Symposium on adolescence. *Pediatr. Clin. North Am., 7:*1-226, 1960.

O'Brien, R. *et al.*: *Body Measurements of American Boys and Girls for Garment and Pattern Construction.* Washington, D.C. U. S. Govt. Printing Office, 1941.

Park, E. A.: Bone growth in health and disease. *Arch. Dis. Child., 29:*269-281, 1954.

Pyle, S. I. *et al.*: Patterns of skeletal development in the hand. *Pediatrics, 24:*886, 1959.

Stuart, H. C.: Normal growth and development during adolescence. *N Engl J. Med., 234:*666, 693, 732, 1946.

Tanner, J. M.: *Growth at Adolescence.* Springfield, Thomas, 1956.

Watson, E. H. *et al.*: *Growth and Development of Children.* Chicago, Year Book, 1967.

Growth Determinants

The human organism is a self-perpetuating combination of atoms, organized in a highly specific manner and interacting with its environment in such a way as to metabolize, grow, adapt and reproduce. Somehow, appropriate reactions occur at the right places and at the right time in individual cells and in the organism as a whole to produce the eventual result preordained in the DNA coding transmitted in the germ cells. The gradual transition from childhood to adulthood is the resultant of many vectorial forces eventually fusing unto maturity. In childhood, growth is active; the body as a whole increases in bulk. In adolescence, the intense activity of growth attains its peak at the spurt and gradually subsides when growth of the body as a whole ceases. The individual stature has been reached and thereafter there is no addition. Growth is most active before the master activities of gland, muscle and nerve have been established. It is the creative principle of the body, and the results of its action make all other activities possible via controlling forces.

Genetic control affects the response of the end organs to all sorts of stimuli; body shape and size, deposition of fat, and patterns of growth are functions of nature rather than nurture. Genetic factors thus play the leading role in establishing the difference between male and female patterns of growth, timing and intensity of the adolescent growth spurt, the size differential between men and women. Marked advancement of girls over boys in skeletal maturation is due to the belated action of the genes on the Y-chromosome of the male. Secular control of growth is universal. Children are now growing faster than ever before, but they are stopping growth much sooner. At the turn of the century man did not reach his final height until twenty-five years of age; now the age has dropped to twenty or less. A striking feature is the progressive advancement in the timing of the menarche. There is increased superiority of girls over boys in regard to I.Q. at the age of eleven years due to the earlier appearance of the adolescent growth spurt.

Hormonal control regulates every phase of adolescent growth. The growth hormone of the anterior pituitary maintains the normal rate of synthesis of proteins in the body, inhibits the synthesis of fats and the oxidation of carbohydrates. The main effect is on the growth and length of the bone, essential for the proliferation of the cartilage cells of the epiphyseal plates with little effect on the maturation of the skeleton. The amount of growth hormone in the bloodstream reveals a daily rhythm varying inversely with the amount of cortisone secretion, food intake and degree of activity, but a major peak appears during the early stages of sleep. The anterior pituitary also secretes the thyrotrophic hormone which affects growth by stimulating the thyroid gland to secrete thyroxin and triiodothyronine. Curiously enough the pituitary and thyroid glands have little effect on the adolescent growth spurt. Neural control by the hypothalamus maintains an individual on his genetically determined growth curve via interaction with the anterior lobe of the pituitary. The peripheral nervous system also controls growth via the nutritional effect on the structures they supply; a chemical compound is secreted by the nerve cells and liberated at the endings of the nerve fibers.

Neuroendocrine control is initiated by nuclei in the limbic region to stimulate the hypothalamus for links in the circuit of individual behavior and endocrine response. The hypothalamus incites anterior pituitary secretion of hormones via neurohumeral secretions or nerve impulses. The hypophysis and hypothalamus are further regulated by circulating hormones from other glands resulting in cyclic interplay. The hypophyseal trophic hormones stimulate their specific target glands: thyrotropin for the thyroid, ACTH for the adrenal cortex, gonadotropins for the gonads, but the growth hormone acts directly on the somatic tissue stimulating the rate of growth and regulating fat metabolism. In the male, the follicle-stimulating hormone acts on the spermatozoa cells in the testes to promote growth of the seminiferous tubule and produce androgen secretion between Leydig's cells in the testes. In the female, follicle-stimulating hormones promote growth of the graafian follicles and the leutinizing hormone released stimulates the estrogen secretion after ovulation.

The newly formed corpus luteum begins to secrete progesterone following a sudden discharge of leutinizing hormone. Estrogens and androgens thus affect the end-organs, the penis, scrotum, seminal vessels and prostate in the male and the uterus, vagina and breasts in the female and the hair and skin in both. Androgens initially stimulate linear growth and muscle development, but eventually both androgens and estrogens limit the rate of growth but stimulate skeletal maturation unto epiphyseal fusion. Experimentally, the afferent stimulation from the genital system also initiates the neuroendocrine mechanism, depending on the inherent genetic factor and the multiple extrinsic factors. Emotional stress may precipitate or delay menstrual flow, vary the time of ovulation and even alter the rate of growth, while emotional deprivation arrests growth.

Nutritional control is manifest when the marked increase in food intake parallels the rapid adolescent growth spurt. Adequate balanced nutrition is essential for increased body needs of active tissue formation. After a period of malnutrition there is growth acceleration to make up the loss in height and weight, to restore the predicted height when the period of malnutrition is completely compensated. Undernutrition accentuates the normal progress of differential growth. For example, in dietary deprivation, the growth of teeth takes precedence over the growth of bone, and bone growth over soft tissues; the growth of sexual organs at puberty is less suppressed than that of other tissues and organs. Socioeconomic control in children of the upper strata makes them taller than those of unskilled laborers by about two inches during adolescence. It is not solely a matter of food but rather home provision of balanced meals, sufficient exercise and sleep and application of the basic rules of hygiene and health. Children in large families are usually smaller and lighter than children in small families because of the lack of individual care, feeding and devotion.

Climatic control does the most where man does the least. Growth in height is faster in the spring than in the autumn by a factor of two and one-half times, while growth in weight is about five times more in the autumn than in the spring. Children tend to grow in the earlier part of the year and fill out in the latter part, though each individual has his own hormonal rhythm of growth. Each race varies in stature according to the climate of his origin. The tallest whites live where winters are cold and wet, as in Scandinavia; while the tallest Australian aborigines thrive under tropical monsoons. There may be geographic effects on height and weight but other forces supersede the meteorological conditions.

Structural Growth

Height in early adolescence increases progressively to the maximum increment in mid-adolescence and decreases gradually during late adolescence when all growth ceases in boys by seventeen and three-fourths years ± ten months; and in girls by sixteen and one-half years ± thirteen months. The timing of the onset of accelerated growth accounts for the extreme differences in size of different youths of the same age. The spurt starts earlier in girls than in boys at about eight to nine years of age, catching up with and passing boys, hence they are often taller and heavier at eleven to thirteen years of age. But boys soon enter a phase of rapid development surpassing the girls unto maturity because both the intensity and duration of the growth spurt is greater in the male than in the female. Ultimate height depends upon the rate of growth at the age when the growth spurt starts and the age when epiphyseal fusion occurs. The adolescent is taller today than a century ago because of the acceleration of maturing processes; the growth spurt is sooner, the rate of growth greater, and the maximal height is attained earlier. Youth matures four months earlier each decade, hence the adult height is reached two years younger than two generations ago.

Height acceleration is about 2.5 cm increase per decade. The skeletal proportions are modified so that the length of the lower extremities equals that of the sitting height in late adolescence. The thorax becomes wider and the pelvis narrower in boys in contrast with girls in whom the reverse maintains. The lower portion of the head grows, with the nose and chin taking the lead and the forehead appearing small by contrast. Myopia increases in adolescence with disproportionate growth of the eyeballs. The developmental status or bone age of an adolescent is determined from roentgenograms. It is a more reliable criterion of biological age than chronological age in predicting a youth's height and evaluating the adequacy of his sexual maturity. In boys, the spurt of growth begins when the skeletal age reaches fourteen years, and in girls, the growth spurt and menarche occur at an earlier bone age but growth ceases when the epiphyses fuse. Strenuous sports should be avoided in boys thirteen to fifteen years of age because serious injury may result from a sudden pull on the epiphysis before fusion.

Facial growth involves the skull vault and orbit related to the nervous system, while facial growth before the base of the skull parallels the rate of growth of the masticatory muscles. The base of the skull is formed in cartilage and growth may continue at the joints between ethmoid, sphenoid, and occipital bones until age twenty-five, when the cartilaginous plate between the occipital and sphenoid bones is obliterated. The growth in the length of the skull is in the plate which pushes the mandible forward. The face grows simultaneously with the development of the jaws and nasopharynx, delaying the permanent facial form until twenty-five years. Its increase in uprightness during growth is due to reduction in the angle of the mandible from 140 degrees in early childhood to 120 degrees in adolescence. Indeed, the mandible is the site of maximal growth activity during the adolescent growth spurt.

Musculature designed for mobility increases rapidly in both sexes, especially in males. Somatic muscles adapt the body to its external environment. Visceral muscles adjust the internal environment with motive power in digestion, circulation, secretion and excretion. Muscles are equally essential for limiting movement. Muscles grow in boys to peak strength between thirteen and sixteen years, and in girls at twelve and one-half years, a year prior to the menarche. Boys excel girls two to fourfold in strength by seventeen years as a result of greater muscle mass. Most of the weight increase in the second phase of the bimodal weight gain is due to increase in skeletal growth and musculature and to some fat deposition. Motor skills increase with motor strength but balance increases continuously with age. There is no such thing as an overgrown, clumsy age unless the clumsy adolescent was a clumsy child. There is a year's lag between achieving body size and developing full muscular power so that a youth should not be subjected to pressure beyond his capacity but controlled exercises stimulate muscle development.

Skin is the seat of external and internal forces in adolescence, the site of active metabolic processes, the special sense organ par excellence creating inhibitory interaction over great surface areas of the body. The whole of the surface of the body is covered by a layer of skin, even the transparent cornea of the eye is overlaid by a continuous layer of modified skin. It is the sensuous mind in skin of microscopic intercellular intensity which makes human contacts by touching pleasant, painful or revolting. The sexual touch of the hand can drive evil spirits out of the heart or create internal turmoil. The laying of the hand establishes communion between two beings for real understanding. There is no conception of youth's mind which has not at first been begotten upon the organs of sense. Youth is astonished at thought but sensation is equally wonderful.

Subcutaneous fat is markedly increased in early adolescence before the growth spurt. It leads to emotional problems giving boys a configuration incorrectly considered hypogonadism since their maturation comes much earlier. After the growth spurt, the increment in body fat deposition decreases again in boys but subcutaneous fat continues to deposit at a greater rate in girls. The second marked increase in weight follows the growth in height. The skin reveals an increase in sebaceous secretion marked in the nasolabial folds in acne. The primary lesion is the comedo which becomes secondarily infected with pus formation. The sweat glands in the axillary, anogenital and palmoplantar regions become hyperactive with consequent hyperhidrosis.

Growth Spurt

Adolescence produces sudden rises in the steady rate of increase in height with little difference between the average heights of boys and girls. The long quiescent interval before the spurt allows time for brain maturation. The spurt begins about ten and one-half to eleven years in girls and twelve and one-half to thirteen years in boys, for about two to two and one-half years with wide variations. Girls gain about six and one-half inches with the peak velocity at twelve years of age. Boys gain about eight inches, mostly from trunk growth, with the peak velocity at fourteen years of age, growing about four inches a year. At the end of the spurt there is a marked slowing of growth, girls reaching 98 percent of their final height by sixteen and one-half years and boys not until seventeen and one-half. Girls become taller and heavier than boys at about eleven years while boys overtake girls in height by fourteen years and become heavier much later. The earlier, feebler growth spurt in girls accounts for the smaller stature of women compared to men, since boys and girls are about the same height before the spurt.

Weight measurement is complicated by several difficulties. Height in the morning is greater than in the evening because the width of the intervertebral discs becomes compressed by the gravitational strain imposed by the upper part of the body during the day. Height is altered by pelvic posture and vertebral column and controlled by muscle tension. Height should thus be measured at the same time of the day by the same person to minimize systemic errors in technique. Height prediction is possible by the second birthday when the child has joined the genetic curve which determines height. Predictive reliability is high from three years to the adolescent spurt with a peak at age eight years for girls and ten years for boys. Such predictions have personal, social and vocational applicability.

The adolescent growth spurt is apparent only by plotting gain in physical characteristics as a function of chronological age. The teenager not only becomes taller but grows at a faster rate determined by genetic inheritance, dietary adequacy and balance, optimal medical care, and other environmental provisions. It is risky to evaluate youth's growth in terms of group averages. Growth does not proceed at the same rate for all body parts; for example, height is not a unitary measure but a composite of gains in leg length and trunk length, each of which grow at different rates and attain a maximum length at different times. A valid indicator of overall physical maturity is to compare x-rays of bone structure with normative data of bone ossification. Skeletal age has its own base line, hence the raw score is the ratio indicating percentage rather than amount of ossification.

Size, strength and stamina of boys are prized in our culture among peers of both sexes, while form, femininity and bloom of girls are equally appreciated by society and deviates frowned upon. But the social assets of early maturation may be offset by psychological liabilities. The early maturer's acceptance of an immediately gratifying social role may foster an identity that precludes further experimentation in different social roles to discover and develop latent abilities. Delay or failure of maturation and/or precocious or uneven maturation are causes for concern to both boys and girls. Early maturers feel self-confident, independent, and adaptable, become prize athletes and student body presidents, while late maturers feel inadequate, rejected and dominated. Cognitively, the late maturer appears better prepared to cope with the demands of maturation, achieving a more flexible autonomous insightful adaptation.

Adolescents are ever anxious about physical development and personal appearance, manifest by compulsive cleanliness, long hours before the mirror, fixation on clothes, comparative evaluation of poor ensembles. The anxiety may reverse itself by sloppiness and neglect as a gesture of despair about unattractiveness, revolt against keeping up appearances or abidance by the raiment of a hippy group to whom the adolescent owes his allegiance. Adolescent anxieties are exploited by commercial interests which make large claims about the magic road to attractiveness, love and popularity by using the right cosmetics, pills and nutrients.

Body Build

The riddle of form is the fundamental riddle of body organization. The entire body and all its component parts grow at varying rates producing striking changes in bodily proportions. The relation between one part of the body and the body as a whole is described by equation $y = bx^k$ where y is the size of one part and x that of another, and b and x are constants. It quantitates the relation between sitting and standing height, arm and trunk length, and so on. New values for b and k become necessary for most paired comparisons. The relation between one part and another of the growing body is ever changing with age. Sitting height increases at adolescence much more rapidly than stature as a whole though it keeps pace with height during childhood.

The dimensions of the head are in advance of the trunk, the trunk in advance of the limbs; and at all ages, the more peripheral parts of the limbs are in advance of the central parts. In the adolescent spurt, the hands and feet accelerate first, then the calf and forearms, then the hips and chest, and finally the shoulders. Last to accelerate is the length of the trunk and the depth of the chest. There is about one year between the peak for the lower limb length and trunk length. The hands and feet are large in relation to the rest of the body, a continuous source of transient anatomical embarrassment to the adolescent. The spurt in trunk length is relatively greater than that in the lower limbs so that more of the increase in height in the adolescent derives from the trunk than from the lower limbs. And the foot stops growing early, before almost all other parts of the skeleton.

The bones of the face grow faster than those of the cranial vault so that the adolescent face emerges from under the skull. The profile becomes straighter and the bone more projecting, especially in boys. Later, in the adolescent spurt, there is laterality rather than a linearity because the limb growth which started first exhausts itself first. The child who shoots up like a beanpole fills himself out in the later stages of the growth spurt. The clavicle which thrusts the shoulder out from the trunk is one of the last bones of the body to stop growing. Slow maturing adolescents tend to be long-legged and slender-hipped at maturity, while fast maturers become broader and more stocky.

The sex differentials in the skeleton are striking. The greater growth of the male shoulder is obviously related to the greater use of the more powerful muscles induced by gonadal hormones, while the differential growth of the female pelvis which makes it wider and roomier than the male pelvis is obviously related to the needs of child-bearing. The male forearm is longer in relation to height than the female forearm. The female index finger is usually longer than the ring finger. Fat deposit in the female at adolescence produces marked alteration in body shape, while fat accumulation in the breasts protects the glands under ovarian hormone control.

Physical types reflect the body build in action. This is a world of bodies, each body with a revealing constitution, each body pushing with a terrible power, each body reacting with its own unrest. There is more wisdom in the body than in deepest philosophy. The variety of shapes and sizes presented by the human body are correlated qualitatively and quantitatively with different temperaments and diseases. Measurements of various parts of the body are reduced by factor analysis to delineate each type of disease susceptibility. One system gives androgeny rating to the shape of the adult body in terms of sexual differences. For example, the male has a low waist while the female has a marked one; the male a wide space between the legs, while the female has a small one; and the hair and fat distribution differ markedly in both sexes.

Sheldon's system of constitutional types has clinical significance. The endomorph is characteristically round with round head, large abdomen, fatty arms and thighs and thin wrists and ankles. His body measures more from front to back than from side to side. The mesomorph has strong shoulders and chest, a transversely lying heart and muscular arms and legs, but little subcutaneous fat. The ectomorph is thin and narrow with little muscle, little subcutaneous fat, thin arms and legs. His heart lies vertically, his skin surface is large, and his nervous system extensive. His adolescent spurt takes place a year later than that of the mesomorph. Each physical type reveals its characteristic temperament that affects the personal life, vocation, and disease susceptibility.

The cerebral type tends to think his way through life, withdraws for inner concentration, minimizes bodily enjoyment and shrinks from excessive activity. It is a difficult way, a lonely climb, and a slippery foothold for enjoying the view when he reaches the top. The visceral type feels his way, performs a bacchic dance through life, up hill and down dale, with quick senses and storm-swift feet ever ready to pause for wine, women and song. The muscular type marches through life with muscles tense, eyes aggressively set on the enemy, never stopping to meditate or to feel, becoming easily demoralized once he relaxes into a life of feeling. Various combinations of these fundamental types prevail with pure forms impossible; relatively pure, rare; and a balance between the three, singular.

Postural patterns reveal body architecture and mental image. The erect posture is not an unmixed blessing with advantages and liabilities. It frees the hands for coordination with the brain stimulated to increase in size and mobilizes the eyes for action. The stance is a precarious equilibrium maintained by CNS with reflexes and controls, straining the vertebral column and the bones and joints of the lower limbs. Violent exercises may strain the ankles; prolonged standing, the arches of the feet; breathing hampered with the weight of the chest wall raised against gravity. Thoracic and abdominal viscera descend, the anterior abdominal wall is weakened, and the pelvis remains primitive. The brain above the heart is deprived of adequate blood supply, hence the postural fainting with sudden rising.

The center of gravity of the adolescent is about half of the total height from the floor, higher in males than in females. The line of gravity alters constantly according to stance. Faulty posture is due to the tilt of the pelvis in relation to the horizontal plane. The pelvic tilt is determined by the postural pull of the muscles of the back, abdomen and thighs and is influenced by the way the individual stands persistently. A tense habit of standing increases the tilt so that the pelvis rotates forward on the thighs, carries the lumbar spine forward and with it the center of gravity. The body compensates with the upper part thrusting backward to increase the lumbar curvature. The neck is held stiff, the chin tucked to maintain the horizontal gaze of the eyes. The slack posture causes the pelvic tilt to decrease, the center of gravity to pass backward and the head and thorax thrust forward in compensation producing thoracic curvature.

Poor posture is temporary in adolescence with bones growing more rapidly than muscles. But a boy who lacks confidence slinks with his head down and a girl conscious of breast enlargement slumps forward. Each must be taught good body mechanics to make them look better and feel better. It means body balance not just a shift of the head, shoulders or abdomen attained by a few mirror demonstrations. Round shoulders is a failure of the muscles of the shoulder girdle to hold the scapula back towards the spine. Conversely, high-heeled shoes tip body weight forward and may produce pain in the neck. Postural deformity may be hereditary or acquired and become manifest in adolescence with the weight increase at the time of the growth spurt, not accompanied by a corresponding increase in the postural muscles, especially in girls.

Maturation Indices

Deviations in the growth of the skeleton produce developmental patterns: the early maturer who is tall in childhood but will not be tall in adulthood, the early maturer who is genetically tall throughout childhood and destined to be a tall adult; the late maturer who is short but will eventually attain average stature; the late developer, genetically short in stature; the ill-defined individual who starts puberty much earlier or later than usual and may turn out to be much taller or shorter than predicted; and the average adolescent. Mental and emotional development are much more closely linked with radiological and dental age than with chronological age. The adolescent considered advanced or retarded physically will reveal parallel features mentally. Adolescents quick to mature physically score higher I.Q.s than those of the same age who have not yet reached the same physical development, but the differential wanes after full maturation of both groups.

The youth who develops late may lag not only in height and weight but also in intelligence and motor skills. He does poorly in school and in athletics, feels rejected and becomes rebellious and aggressive. On the other hand, the one who develops early is in a bad psychological state for he is physically bigger than his colleagues and cannot fit into the educational system or the social mores. Attainment of an adult body and sexual maturity before attainment of economic independence produces an uncomfortable situation aggravated by enforced educational demands.

Mental age is measured by performance tests of arithmetical, verbal, logical and other specific abilities. The mental age is thus an index of the maturation of mind which increases at a rate depending upon intrinsic and environmental factors. The mental status can lag behind unless the child has the opportunity to sharpen his wits on problems, to acquire experience in the art of everyday living and to develop greater responsibility as an independent being. The intrinsic factors alone do not determine the mental age without specific enhancement by external forces. What is innate may never come to pass unless brought to the fore by training and experience. Mental development reaches maturity between fifteen and twenty-five years of age, but intellectual performance continues to improve throughout life by knowledge, training and experience, even though the mental capacity to deal with intellectual material does not increase. The know-what and the know-how enable an individual to function more smoothly, whatever the intellectual level attained.

Physiological age reflects the biochemical changes directly related to alteration in size. For example, heart rate is inversely proportional to body size. The filtration rate of the renal glomeruli attains adult levels at age three, but blood pressure continues to rise not only throughout growth but also throughout life. The BMR falls rapidly from age six to twenty and gradually throughout life with a transient rise during the adolescent spurt. The sexual differential accounts for many of the biochemical changes. Girls show a spurt in systolic blood pressure earlier than boys. Mouth temperature reaches adult readings earlier in girls, but it continues to fall by another one-half degree in boys. Red cell count and blood volume of boys diverge from the figures for girls during the adolescent spurt. A valuable index of maturation is the ratio of creatine to creatinine in the urine which falls progressively after age fourteen and one-half years under hormonal influence. Girls maturing early have a lower ratio than those of the same chronological age maturing late, hence the ratio is valuable along with skeletal and radio-logical data in determining the level of maturity.

Sexual age in the male begins with the earliest sign of puberty: growth of the testicles shortly after hypothalamic signal initiating the sexual process. Mitotic figures abound in the seminiferous tubules, spermatozoa begin to form and testosterone appears in the urine. After hormone production from the testes and supra-renals, the penis enlarges in size, accompanied by changes in the larynx, skin and hair distribution on the body. Rating of sexual maturation of the secondary sexual characteristics utilizes a one to five scale for hair, breast and genital growth. The sexual spurt is subject to the same wide variations as the growth spurt, for some boys of fourteen may be practically mature sexually while others have not begun their sexual spurt. Growth acceleration of the larynx does not occur until termination of the penile spurt with direct testosterone stimulation of the laryngeal cartilage cells and associated soft parts. Pubic hair occurs before the spurt in height; facial and ancillary hair does not appear for two years after pubic hair. The apocrine sweat glands of the axilla and genital regions increase in number and are activated at puberty. The scrotal skin darkens and the prostate and seminal vessels enlarge concurrently with the penis.

The first internal sign of puberty in the female is increase in the size of the ovaries and the quantity of estrogen excretion in the urine is the index of ovarian activity. The first external sign of female puberty is enlargement of the breasts which precedes the peak of the adolescent spurt. The growth of the uterus and vagina accelerates simultaneously while pubic hair makes its appearance. The vaginal epithelium thickens and accumulates glycogen while the bacterial flora in the vagina produces the acid reaction. Sexual age may be discerned from several stages in sex development. Onset of menstruation can be timed with accuracy after the peak of the growth spurt corresponding to the period of maximal deceleration of growth. Early menstrual cycles may not involve ovulation, hence full sexual maturation may be delayed for a year or two after menstruation has begun; conversely, cyclic liberation of ova may occur in girls much earlier than the onset of menstruation. The age at which the menarche occurs is more closely related to radiologic age than to chronological age. Menstruation according to chronological age occurs between ten and sixteen years of age, while according to radiological age from twelve to fourteen and one-half years: the time of fusion of the epiphyses of the terminal phalanges of the fingers.

Bone age assesses radiological age for physical maturation better than chronological age or body measurements. The wrist and hand are most commonly used because of their large number of centers of ossification. As a rule the rest of the skeleton behaves similarly except in bone disorders. Leg length accelerates first, followed by hip width, chest breadth, shoulder breadth, trunk length and chest depth. The foot has its small acceleration six months before the calf; it is the first part of the skeleton to cease growing. The calf length accelerates before the thigh, the forearm six months ahead of the upper arm. Male legs are longer because the boys' growth spurt occurs later than the girls'. Individual variation in maturation of the skeleton is so consistent that it is quite possible for a child at one stage of development to be widely separated from the median maturity picture without implying any deleterious effect on his future. But if serial x-rays at six-month intervals show a consistent deviation from the median, the matter has to be regarded very seriously. If the hand does not reflect true indications of the growth progress, radiographs of other regions should be taken. Skeletal maturation usually parallels skeletal growth until the epiphyses close. The radiological age of girls is in advance of that of boys by more than 20 percent.

REFERENCES

Atkinson, R. M. *et al.*: Biographical and psychological features in extraordinary fatness. *Psychosom. Med., 29:*121-33, 1967.

Bach, W. G.: Teen-age patients. *Hospitals, 44:*51-3, 1970.

Bayer, L. M. *et al.*: *Growth Diagnosis: Selected Methods for Interpreting and Predicting Physical Development from One Year to Maturity.* Chicago, University Chicago Press, 1959.

Bayley, N.: Individual patterns of development. *Child Dev., 27:*45-74, 1956.

Blizzard, R. M.: The differential diagnosis and treatment of short stature at adolescence. *J. Iowa Med. Soc.*, 54:219-28, 1964.

Boswell, J. I. Jr. *et al.:* Hyperthyroid children: individual and family dynamics. *J. Am. Acad. Child Psychiatry*, 6:64-85, 1967.

Brain, Lord: *Speech Disorders.* London, Butterworth, 1965.

Breeling, J. L.: Adolescent nutrition. *Ill. Med. J.*, 140:217-20, 1971.

Brozek, J. (Ed.): *Human Body Composition.* Oxford, 1965.

Bullard, D. M. Jr.: *Response of the Child to Chronic Physical Disability.* Symposium on Chest Disorders in Children. New York, Am. Physical Therapy Assoc., 1968.

Bullough, W. S.: *The Evolution of Differentiation.* London, 1967.

Cheek, E. B. (Ed.): *Human Growth.* Philadelphia, Saunders, 1968.

Clark, W. E.: *The Tissues of the Body.* Oxford, 1965.

Clifford, E.: Body satisfaction in adolescence. *Percept. Mot. Skills, 33:*119-25, 1971.

Daly, M. J.: Physical and psychological development of the adolescent female. *Clin. Obstet. Gynecol.,* 9:711-21, 1966.

Dwyer, J. T. *et al.:* Adolescent Dieters. *Am. J. Clin. Nutr.,* 20:1045-56, 1967.

Dwyer, J.: Variations in physical appearance during adolescence. *Postgrad. Med., 41:*91, 1967.

Escalona, S. K.: *The Roots of Individuality.* Chicago, Aldine, 1968.

Fairbank, T.: *An Atlas of General Affections of the Skeleton.* Edinburgh, Livingstone, 1951.

Finn, J. A. *et al.:* Left-handedness: a study of its relation to opposition. *J. Proj. Tech. Pers. Assess.,* 32:49-52, 1968.

Forbes, G. B.: Growth of the lean body mass during childhood and adolescence. *J. Pediatr.,* 64:822, 1964.

Fried, R. *et al.:* Socio-economic factors accounting for growth failure in children living in institutions. *J. Pediatr.,* 33:444, 1948.

Frish, M. *et al.:* Overweight in adolescents—a complex problem. *Ann. Pediat.,* 12:234-45, 1966.

Gardner, L. I. (Ed.): *Endocrine and Genetic Diseases of Childhood.* Philadelphia, Saunders, 1969.

Goodman, H. G. *et al.:* Growth and growth hormone. *N. Engl. J. Med.,* 278:57, 1968.

Goodman, P.: *Growing Up Absurd.* New York, Random House, 1960.

Greulich, W. W. *et al.:* *Somatic and Endocrine Studies of Puberal and Adolescent Boys.* Washington, D.C., Soc. Research Child Development, Monograph, Vol. 7, No. 3, 1942; *Radiographic Atlas of Skeletal Development of the Hand and Wrist,* 2d ed. Stanford, Stanford Univ. Press, 1959.

Hall, P. F.: *Gynecomastia.* Sydney, Australia Med. Publishing, 1959.

Hammar, S. L.: The obese adolescent. *J. Sch. Health,* 25:246-9, 1965.

Held, F. P.: Anatomy, physiology and pharmacology of the adolescent. In Cooke, R. E.: *The Biologic Basis of Pediatric Practice.* New York, McGraw-Hill, 1968.

Hoch, P. H. *et al.* (Eds.): *Psychopathology of Communication.* New York, Grune & Stratton, 1958.

Holt, K. S.: The handicapped in society. *J. R. Coll. Gen. Pract.,* 17 (Suppl. 2):23-8, 1969.

Hsia, D. Y-Y: *Inborn Errors of Metabolism,* 2d ed. Chicago, Year Book Medical Publishers, 1966.

Hulka, J. F.: The mature minor. *N. Engl. J. Med.,* 278:1296, 1968.

Hutcheson, B. R.: Money can't buy maturity. *Int. J. Psychiatry,* 4:312-3, 1967.

Jacobs, D. *et al.:* Obesity: Prevention. *J.A.M.A.,* Vol. 186, Suppl. 27-40, 1963.

Johnson, J.: *Nutritional Studies in Adolescent Girls and Their Relation to Tuberculosis.* Springfield, Thomas, 1953.

Jones, M. C.: The later careers of boys who were early-or-late-maturing. *Child Devel.,* 28:113-28, 1957; Psychological correlates of somatic development. *Child Develop.,* 36:899-911, 1965.

Kagan, J. *et al.: Birth to Maturity.* New York, John Wiley, 1962.

Kestenberg, J. S.: Phases of adolescence. *J. Am. Acad. Child Psychiatry,* 7: 108-51, 1968.

Knight, J. A.: The profile of the normal adolescent. *Ann. Allergy,* 25:129-36, 1967.

Kugelmass, I. N.: *Biochemical Diseases, (Chemical Pediatrics).* Springfield, Thomas, 1964.

Kuhlen, R. A.: *The Psychology of Adolescent Development.* New York, Harper & Row, 1952.

Lane, R. E.: Gynecologic profile of the late teenager. *Ill. Med. J.,* 135:582-5, 1969.

Langer, L. O. *et al.:* Achondroplasia. *Am. J. Roentgengol.,* 100:12, 1967.

Leverett, H. M.: Vision test performance of school children. *Am. J. Ophthalmol.,* 44:508-10, 1957.

Leverton, R. M.: The paradox of teen-age nutrition. *J. Am. Diet Assoc.,* 53: 6, 1968.

Lourie, R. S.: Diagnosis in adolescent problems. *Clin. Proc. Child Hosp. DC,* 23:33-40, 1967.

Marshall, W. A. *et al.:* Growth and physiological development during adolescence. *Ann. Rev. Med.,* 19:283-300, 1968.

McKusnick, V. A. *et al.:* The genetic mucopolysaccharidoses. *Med.,* 44:445, 1965.

Meredith, H. V.: Body size of contemporary youth in different parts of the world. *Monogr. Soc. Res. Child Dev.,* 34:1-120, 1969.

Meyer, J. E.: Anorexia nervosa of adolescence. *Br. J. Psychiatry, 118:*539-42, 1971.

Nicholson, A. B. *et al.:* Indices of physiological maturity: derivation and interrelationships. *Child Dev., 24:*3-28, 1953.

Odell, W. D.: Isolated deficiencies of anterior pituitary hormone. *J.A.M.A., 197:*176, 1966.

Offer, D. *et al.:* A longitudinal study of normal adolescent boys. *Am. J. Psychiatry, 126(7):*917-924, 1970.

Phelps, W. M. *et al.: The Diagnosis and Treatment of Postural Defects.* Springfield, Thomas, 1956.

Ramsay, R. W.: Speech patterns and personality. *Lang. Speech, 11:*54-63, 1968.

Richardson, F.: Stature and personality. (Bonaparte N) *Br. Med. J., 1:*516-7, 1968.

Sanchez, R. C.: Medical care of the adolescent. *J. La. State Med. Soc., 118:* 506-10, 1966.

Seckel, H. P. G.: *Bird-headed Dwarfs.* Springfield, Thomas, 1960.

Shapiro, L. R. *et al.:* Teenagers: their body size and shape, food, and activity. *J. Sch. Health, 37:*166-70, 1967.

Silver, H. K. *et al.:* Deprivation dwarfism. *J. Pediatr., 70:*317, 1967.

Sinclair, D.: *Human Growth After Birth.* London, Oxford Univ. Press, 1969.

Smith, D. W.: Compendium on shortness of stature. *J. Pediatr., 70:*463, 1967.

Spivack, G. *et al.:* Adolescent symptomatology. *Am. J. Ment. Defic., 72:*74-95, 1967.

Tanner, J. M.: *Growth at Adolescence.* Springfield, Thomas, 1962.

Thompson, J. A.: Factors affecting growth in man. *Scott. Med. J., 15:*272, 1970.

Warren, W.: The adolescent patient. *Guys Hosp. Rep., 119:*337-46, 1970.

Watson, E. H. *et al.: Growth and Development of Children.* Chicago, Year Book, 1967.

Whitnall, E. *et al.: The Deaf Child.* London, Heinemann Med. Books, 1964.

Widdowson, E. M.: Mental contentment and physical growth. *Lancet, 1:* 1316, 1951.

Wilkins, L.: *The Diagnosis and Treatment of Endocrine Disorders in Childhood and Adolescence.* Springfield, Thomas, 1960.

Wright, B. A.: *Physical Disability, a Psychological Approach.* New York, Harper & Row, 1960.

Youlton, R. *et al.:* Growth and growth hormone. *Pediatrics, 43:*989, 1969.

Young, C. M. *et al.:* Body composition of pre-adolescent and adolescent girls. *J. Am. Diet Assoc., 53:*25-31, 1968.

Young, H. B. *et al.:* Evaluation of physical maturity of adolescence. *Dev. Med. Child Neurol., 10:*338-348, 1968.

CHAPTER III

MENTAL IMMATURITY

Mind is the great lever of all things;
human thought is the process by which
adolescent ends are ultimately answered.

The mind of man comprises four historical layers—the animal mind, the child mind, the savage mind, and the civilized mind. The retardate lacks the upper mental layer and much of the other layers following developmental failure of biological maturation that reduces personal abilities and restricts social intercourse. His consciousness is greatly deprived of awareness, thinking, knowing, focusing attention, planning action, interpreting present experience and perceiving the world about him. The retarded mind may have some strength to bewail its feebleness, even though the retardate is oblivious of his failings. The feeble ego may have the psychological capacity through which consciousness is somewhat organized and integrated, through which his being is somewhat set in motion physically and mentally, and through which his adaptive thought and behavior is so poorly achieved. The retarded mind thus becomes a dangerous weapon if youth knows not how or when or where to use it discreetly; it becomes a strange machine which combines the materials offered to it in the most astonishing ways for aberrant behavior; it becomes more intuitive than logical and comprehends little to coordinate without individualized intensive training. After all, it is the mind which is really alive and sees things, yet it hardly sees anything without effective instruction. The whole secret of the teachers' force lies in the conviction that retardates are reversible.

The tempo of the adolescent retardate makes him reason more slowly, learn more slowly, memorize more slowly, move more slowly, and respond more slowly than the normal youth. Yet he walks firmer and more secure up hill than down. It points to the fact that the ultimate measure of the retardate is not where he stands in moments of comfort and convenience at home, but where he stands in times of stress and strain in the world without. The moment he emerges beyond the home, peace and security drop out of consciousness, for the only psychic equilibrium is in the degree of fulfillment possible for him to realize. The only peace, the only security is in some fulfillment. The kind related to the world may be trivial, but even being related to an insignificant pattern is immensely preferable to being alone at home. Life without some absorbing interest is hell—for him joy consists in forgetting life. He is most aware of his role; he never occupies the middle of his cage; his whole being surges toward the bars. His view of life is hateful as a spectator but absorbing as a participant. Knowledge of what is possible in participation of any kind in life is the beginning of some semblance of happiness with the gradual growth of intellectual development, learning ability, social competence and rational behavior. The retardate is not the sum of the little he has already, but rather the sum of what he does not yet have.

Lack of Intellectual Development

Adolescent retardates reveal individualized characteristics of behavior interwoven with emotional disturbance, physical disability, and neurological defect—all reflecting genetic errors. Every defect and infirmity must be paid for in this hard and precarious world of the poor, unemployed, deprived, malnourished, and uneducated where retardation abounds. All attempts to explain the personality of the retardate by extrapolation from normal adolescents are fallacious. Some maintain that the retardate is socially incompetent with developmental arrest at maturity; others, that the retardate has slowness to learn as the common denominator; still others, that the retardate behavior is related to disturbed interpersonal relations and the nature of the emotional disorders is not different from that of the normal adolescent. Actually, the retardate is difficult to characterize by specific criteria or overt stigmata as in disease. Indeed, the personality patterns are more unique than ever observed among deviates. The hardest thing to cope with among adolescents is not selfishness or vanity or deceitfulness but sheer stupidity—

congenital or acquired. To serve a dull mind is like crying in the wilderness, planting water lilies on dry land or whispering in the ear of the deaf. When you point to the moon, the dullard looks at the finger. Fortunately, he is blessed with some common sense which is more useful to him than exalted sense, because a little knowledge requires a lot of common sense to apply it.

The dullard is an outcast in the world, ready physically but no place to go mentally; confused emotionally, and inept socially. He must choose between boredom and torment, and so he yields to the former until it becomes the most sublime of emotions; it thus confirms the biologist's contention that man is the only animal that can be bored. The dynamics of his psyche are similar to that of the normal adolescent with secret pleasures and ubiquitous yearnings, with deep-seated guilt and few outlets for sublimation, with craving for affect and limited means for reciprocity. He is frightened by masturbation, frustrated by heterosexual stimulation and distressed about homosexual play. He shows unresolved dependence upon his family, limited repertoire of social skills, and primitive expression of fantasy. Assessment of the intellectual capacities unravels the basis of excessive emotionality, impaired judgment, aberrant activity, limitations not always obvious when the subnormality is mild, the youth outgoing, the behavior well-mannered.

Three groups of mental retardates are observed amongst adolescents. One reveals physiological retardation, educable I.Q. 80 to 50, arising from sociocultural deprivation, undereducation and polygenic organic factors, but needs guidance when under unusual social or economic stress. Another group is trainable I.Q. 50 to 30, arising from systemic, neurological defects and/or polygenic organic forces. A third group, I.Q. 30 to 0, pathologically retarded adolescents, distinct from the adolescent population that must be supervised *in toto* in daily life. Fortunately, the physiologic group with I.Q. over 50 outnumber the pathologic group by a ratio of 10:1, which poses a problem not only for parents but for educators, sociologists and economists. Young adolescents may be tested by the WISC, older adolescents by the WAIS psychometric yardsticks, involving verbal performance and full scale time-consuming I.Q. measures. The Amors' quick screening test is a picture, nonverbal, vocabulary evaluation to detect degrees of mental dysfunction. The visual motor Gestalt test measures perceptive motor organization for revealing minimal brain damage. Draw-a-man measures the nonverbal phase of development which requires relatively normal status. Vineland Social Maturity Scale measures social development for total personality orientation.

The etiologic diagnosis of mental retardation is necessary for planning intelligent therapy, prognosis, and counselling. The diagnostic work-up should be discussed with parents on the basis of the initial impression formulated at one time rather than piecemeal. History taking and physical examination provide more important information than any single laboratory procedure. The pregnancy, birth, neonatal course, behavior throughout childhood, history of a transmissible neurological disorder throw light on the underlying basis of the retardation. The presence of a congenital malformation in other organ systems always raises the suspicion of a nervous system anomaly. Skull x-rays rarely yield useful diagnostic information. Metabolic screening tests on urine and blood uncover rare inborn errors in metabolism. EEG patterns are characteristic of high and low intelligence. Dull subjects do not have significant differences in the electrical activity of the two hemispheres of the brain, while bright youths show marked differences. Buccal smear chromatin studies can be performed easily and painlessly when the etiology of the retardation is obscure. Many chromatin-positive and chromatin-negative females are found to be mentally retarded.

The diagnostic profile of a mental retardate should illuminate the ways and means of attaining the fullest maturation possible. If the objectives of the case study are limited to standard diagnostic classification, the retardate will become lost in anonymity. The clinical goal is to understand the retardate as a maturing being, to uncover the dynamics of his way of life, to define his inner and outer needs, and to determine the kinds of help he requires to become whatever he is capable of being. It will take three times longer to train him than the normal, but it can be

done, despite limits of competence. There is no mentally retarded adolescent whose measured intelligence and physiological
impairment are beyond some significant increment of functional
and adaptive gain. Every adolescent, normal and retarded, mature
or immature, rich or poor, falls heir to anxiety. It is the physician's responsibility to identify the extent to which ego pathology
vitiates progress, constricts motivation, embarrasses learning behavior, distorts perception, impairs abstract thinking and blocks
functioning.

How does the retardate secure the information from the world
about him so essential for his adaptation to it and his survival in
it? Outreaching mental mechanisms like antennae search out
the required perceptual information. Only an extremely small
fraction of all the sensory input is actually experienced by the
normal individual. And only an extremely small proportion of
all patterned neuronal activity going on in his brain at any one
time gives rise to conscious experience; though within limits, he
may apparently direct his attention to other neuronal patterns,
which as a consequence are then consciously experienced. Likewise, only an extremely small fraction of the sensory input into
the brain will he recall in the process of memory, even for a few
minutes of short-term memory. Apparently, the neural processes
underlying learning and forgetting, storage and retrieval of memory traces are very, very small with respect to the background
activity of the cerebrum. All human achievements from the lowest to the highest levels are dependent upon them. But in the
mentally retarded, the whole spectre of cerebral dynamics from
input to output approaches the minimal, with input exceeding
the output in mental stimulation.

We therefore investigate systematically the retardate's processes and style of perception; we inquire into how he deals with
what he perceives internally; we examine his memory, his store
of knowledge, his ability to recall. We evaluate, too, his ways of
thinking, his trends of thought, their coherence and relevance;
we judge his intellectual flexibility, his capacity for abstraction,
his abilities in communication. What the retarded can do is
more significant than what he cannot; when he cannot, why can

he not? Special education programs for the adolescent retardate must recognize that he feels inadequate, appears gullible, remains socially awkward; he suffers from body-image disturbance, equilibrium imbalance, abnormal impulse patterns and impaired communication capacity. Consequently, the environment must be warm, not overly permissive, orderly in organization, and consistent in discipline. Boring tasks should be avoided, distractions minimized, extraneous noises limited. Specific techniques help the adolescent overcome perceptual problems by translating abstract concepts into concrete terms. Vocational training should be emphasized and mastery of academic subjects abandoned in preparation for an intellectually undemanding but useful occupation.

Lack of Learning Ability

Adolescents' learning problems reveal residuals of childhood problems at various levels of development. Once the origin of the learning difficulty is determined, correction is directed at the underlying dynamic disorder rather than at the current learning problem. Specific learning disability, especially reading retardation, abounds in boys more than in girls. It may be a primary reading problem reflecting a disturbed pattern of neurologic organization. There is an inability to deal with letters and words as symbols leading to a diminished ability to integrate the meaningfulness of written material. It may be secondary despite a normal capacity to read, because of negativism, anxiety, depression psychosis, limited schooling, or other external influences, or due to brain injury with neurologic deficits and other aphasic difficulties. What youth knows is of little moment; he must be taught how to learn. Everywhere we learn only from those whom we love.

Learning difficulties correlate with specific subject matter which has unconscious meaning related to the individual's personality structure. There may be so much anxiety around a special area that he cannot possibly learn the subject. Occasionally, the adolescent rebellion takes the form of refusing to perform whatever is expected of him. He may learn the subject matter adequately yet refuse to comply with the specific requirements which determine the final grading and thus fail rather than yield. Adolescents whose ego function of cognition is defective cannot learn because they do not have the ego capacity to profit from educational material in a meaningful way. Learning is essential in adolescence for world adaptation and vocational preparation. The adolescent should begin to want to learn skills and develop insight into subject matter. It is a mature kind of learning, impossible if the student is blocked by his own sexual and aggressive impulses. Immature adolescents are motivated to learn only to please others, but it should be continued until a more effective approach is inculcated. Treatment of adolescent learning problems requires elucidation of the difficulty, development of intellectual insight into the dynamic differentiation of school and teacher from home and parents; opportunity for discussion of academic behavior with the medical authority without making learning an arena for the battle between himself and his parents.

Adolescent difficulty at the onset of puberty has its roots in the unresolved conflicts of earlier developmental periods. Early ego failure produces special problems throughout adolescence. The total personality may not be fixated at this point, but some aspects or residues of early developmental problems may persist in the personality makeup. Defects in the autonomous ego process have subsequent effects on learning because painful sensations and defective perceptions interfere with autonomous functions indispensable for progressive ego maturation. Early schizoid traits affect learning in many ways, especially with the use of logic by the intrusion of fantasy. Affective disorders cause withdrawal from the learning scene. Schizoid reactions from adolescent pressures block learning capacity. Sublimation is a determining ego function in early life, evident in latency when all impulses tend to be controlled, but inability to sublimate into learning is an innate deficiency that produces an ego defect.

Passive learners depend on the support or identification with teachers and thus fail to act independently. Such osmotic learners have high intelligence but are unwilling to work. They acquire techniques of getting along with minimal work. But the learning is not integrated with their being. What pious fraud to go to school to please an external force rather than an internal interest and remain on the periphery of school learning to adapt superficially. They play make-believe, pretend to take themselves and everyone else seriously—to love one another, hate one another—but then it isn't true! They don't care at all. Such deceit is the game of warped minds. There is no remedy for human apathy. Love, learning and work—the great harmonizers between youth and the rest of the world—must all be inculcated. The pupil who remembers day to day what he has yet to learn and from month to month what he learned already truly develops a love of learning.

Aggressive learners seek the love of the teacher by attention-getting devices, hand raising, arguing and battling. Aggressive competition with classmates or teacher exposes hostile, competitive attitudes that are displaced from siblings and parents and excessive need for love from inadequate self-esteem. Some aggressive students remain content with failure because they have given up trying to attain the love they want and so have given up learning per se. They want approval desperately and if not forthcoming, suffer depression. Oral sadism takes the form of sarcasm while stubbornness is rooted in anal defiance. Unconscious defiance takes many forms; some adolescents forget assignments; others postpone studying; and many wander into fantasy. Perfection is an obsessive, compulsive technique used without defiance of superego pressures. Learning becomes an end in itself at the gate of knowledge. There is no royal road to learning.

Lack of School Achievement

The mediocre adolescent who does not hope to succeed has already failed. Endowed with small talents, he is not spurred into great ambition and the results are revealing. By their fruits ye shall know them. Academic achievement falls below expectation of intellectual capacity in 10 percent of the adolescent population. The learning disorders are associated with inadequate nutrition, systemic disease, perceptive disorder and predominantly emotional difficulty. There is no inertness, inactivity or laziness

because youth must be doing something or fancy that he is doing something, for in him throbs the creative impulse. We must
recognize school failure early for in the lexicon of youth there
is no such word as fail unless the mind is dull and the body difficult. Formal academic learning begins at six years when the
convergence of physical, emotional and intellectual maturation
confers the capacity for learning. It takes developmental maturity or myelination of associational pathways to fulfill learning
tasks, utilizing symbols to represent concepts. Thought once
awakened does not slumber.

Maturation lag blocks development of human capacity but
maturational forces unfold in response to effective stimulation in
a proper environment. Systemic disorders must be ruled out,
such as vitamin deficiency, anemia, fatigue, anxiety, as well as
visual, auditory and motor coordination difficulties. Each adolescent utilizes his sensual modalities in an individual way with
sensory preferences in the use of these pathways. For example,
some individuals will see the letter of a word as gestalt and comprehend through this mode, while others will rely on hearing a
word pronounced to remember it. These difficulties account for
the two forms of reading approaches used by educators as the
visual and auditory methods respectively. Dyslexia or word blind-
ness produces an inability to understand the written language
with difficulty in reading from left to right, leading to mirror
images and reversal of letters in words. There may be lack of
motor coordination due to cerebral dysfunction and there is poorly established cerebral dominance. Neurological examination is
normal, but there are soft neurological signs disclosing emotional
difficulties, crossed dominance, sensory discrimination and motor
coordination.

Situational problems involve past grading according to age
and capacity. A bright child may be understimulated, spend
time daydreaming and become a behavior problem. A slow
child finds himself forced to compete unsuccessfully and retreats
to daydreams to escape from reality; a fearful child may be threatened by a bully or a gang and thus interfere with attention, concentration and memory. Emotional difficulties may arise from

traumatic experiences during childhood, such as family disruption, separation, accident, hospitalization. Most adolescents with psychological learning difficulties have residual emotional immaturities that interfere with work effort. First, there is the dependent adolescent who remains much younger emotionally, preferring to have things done for him. Then, there is the individual with learning disability who refuses to accommodate to the world around him. Finally, there is the youth who has progressed to a more mature level but remains inhibited, frightened of competition, which generates regrets, envies and hatreds of peers.

Dependent youth has been either infantilized or never stimulated to assume an active role in mastering the world. He is inadequately equipped to assume advanced schooling; he wants rewards without working for them, success without studying; he demands that life take care of him without effort on his part and believes that everyone will love him no matter what he does. Life for the dependent adolescent is full of steep stairs to go up and shaky stairs to totter down, hence the invention of parental banisters. Actually every youth expects somebody or something to help him. And when he finds he must help himself, he cries for liberty and justice. The obstinate youth fails to advance academically because of oppositional attitudes. His constant fear of parental disapproval inhibits his competitive spirit and avoids any aggressive situation that is potentially dangerous. The youth who is swimming against the stream knows the strength of it.

Some adolescents displace home problems on to the school with conscious awareness that the school failure is the most severe form of retaliation within their power against their parents. Other adolescents displace the home struggle on to the school without conscious awareness when the teacher is unconsciously equated with a parent. The overwhelming importance of sexuality or of relationships to overcome feelings of loneliness may relegate little capacity for sublimation. Learning is an ego function whose ultimate purpose is mastery of the environment for survival, but it is necessary as a mode of sublimation of primitive urges, draining off libido anxieties or tensions from conflicts.

Some adolescents have little capacity for sublimation while others remain preoccupied with primitive impulses to such a degree that learning is a drudge devoid of its sublimation function.

MENTAL MATURATION

The brain is the most dynamic of all tissues. Its neurons fire impulses up to 1,000 per second at velocities up to 100 mps. It is always active in sleep and in wakefulness. The mind of man is the recent product of billions of years of cosmic and biological evolution; the most intricate of all works of nature. We are beginning to account for mental powers in terms of this intricate chemical and electrical machinery. The mind directs its attention to one main interest at a time to produce a series of thoughts and considered actions, rather than to strive to deal with everything at once. Attention is the mechanism which decides from moment to moment what we're going to notice and, therefore, what we're going to do. There seems to be a differential filter to protect the central systems from being overloaded. The mind craves continuous excitement, evidenced from the mechanisms of waking, sleeping and dreaming, but at least once a day it is all switched off. The workings of the mind are influenced by body chemistry. If awakening to consciousness is a chemical process, if attention is governed by the flickering action of brain cells, if changes in thought are affected by inculcating hormones, what price mental powers? Yet the will of man can override the most discordant body chemistry. The conscious mind has the most astonishing control over basic bodily function, but there is increasing evidence in favor of determinism against the concept of free will. The direction of the mind is more important than its progress.

Mental Maturation Tests and Measurements

Berko, J. *et al.*: Psycholinguistic research methods. In P. H. Mussen, (Ed.): *Handbook of Research Methods in Child Development.* New York, Wiley, 1960.

Brown, R. *et al.*: Word association and the acquisition of grammar. *Child Dev.*, 31:14, 1960.

Dale, E. *et al.*: *A Formula for Predicting Readability.* The Educational Research Bulletin, Vol. 37, p. 11, 1948.

Elkind, D. *et al.*: Perceptual decentration learning and performance in slow and average readers. *J. Educ. Psychol.*, 56:50, 1965.

Farber, B. *et al.*: *Family Organization and Parent-Child Communications.* Monographs of the Society for Research in Child Development. 1963.

Gesell, A. *et al.*: *Developmental Diagnosis.* New York, Harper, 1941.

Gibson, E. J. *et al.*: The visual cliff. *Sci. Am.*, 202:64, 1960.

Guilford, J. P.: The structure of intellect. *Psychol. Bull.*, 53:267, 1956.

Hammill, D. D. *et al.*: An abstraction test adapted for use with mentally retarded children. *Am. J. Ment. Defic.*, 70:866, 1966.

Hildrent, G. H.: *Introduction to the Gifted.* New York, McGraw-Hill, 1966.

Hunt, J. McV.: *Intelligence and Experience.* New York, Ronald, 1961.

Kagan, J. *et al.*: Information processing in the child. *Psychol. Monogr.*, Vol. 78, No. I., 1964.

Kuhlman, F.: *Tests of Mental Development.* A Complete Scale for Individual Examination. Minneapolis, Educational Test Bureau, 1939.

Lowenfeld, V.: *Your Child and his Art.* New York, Macmillan, 1955.

Luria, A. R.: *The Role of Speech in the Regulation of Normal and Abnormal Behavior.* London, Pergamon Press, 1961.

Parshall, H. W.: A Bible knowledge test for institutionalized mental defectives. *Am. J. Ment. Defic.*, 64:960, 1960.

Piaget, J.: Development and learning. *J. Res. Sci. Teaching*, 3:176, 1964.

Pollack, M. *et al.*: The face-hand test in retarded and non-retarded emotionally disturbed children. *Am. J. Ment. Defic.*, 64:758, 1960.

Radaker, L. D.: The visual imagery of retarded children and the relationship to memory for word forms. *Except. Child.*, 27:524, 1961.

Riggs, M. M. *et al.*: *A Classification System for the Mentally Retarded.* Training School Bulletin, 69, 1952.

Santostefano, S.: Cognitive controls and exceptional states in children. *J. Clin. Psychol.*, 20:213, 1964.

Spradlin, J. E.: Assessment of speech and language of retarded children. The Parsons Language sample. *J. Speech Hear. Disord.*, No. 10, Jan. 1963.

Teahan, J. E.: Future time perspective, optimism and academic achievement. *J. Abnorm. Psychol.*, 57:379, 1958.

Terman, L. *et al.*: *Stanford-Binet Intelligence Scale: Manual for the Third Revision*, Form L-M. Boston, Houghton Mifflin, 1960.

Torrance, E. P.: Education and creativity. In C. W. Taylor (Ed.): *Creativity: Progress and Potential.* New York, McGraw-Hill, 1964.

Williams, W. G.: The adequacy and usefulness of an objective language scale when administered to elementary school children. *J. Educ. Res.* 54:30, 1960.

Witkin, H. A. *et al.: Personality through Perception.* New York, Harper, 1954.

Yerkes, R. M.: Psychological examining in the United States Army. *Mem. Nat. Acad. Sci.,* 15, 1921.

Zeaman, D. *et al.:* The role of attention in retardate discrimination learning. In N. R. Ellis (Ed.): *Handbook of Mental Deficiency.* New York, McGraw-Hill, 1963.

Ziller, R. C. *et al.:* Some correlates of the don't know responses in opinion questionnaires. *J. Soc. Psychol.,* 67:129, 1965.

Mental Abilities

Intelligence is the individual capacity for acquiring facts. It is quickness in seeing things as they are, a native endowment that attains its peak at sixteen years as a multifaceted adaptive capacity that undergoes qualitative reorganization throughout life. It evolves with growing capacity to perceive dynamic processes, original or imitative, in an individual realm of activity, and in social traditions laid down in symbolic forms. Reason is man's faculty for grasping the world by thought, while intelligence is man's ability to manipulate the world with the help of thought. The hereditary component in normal variations of intelligence is determined by a multiplicity of games with small cumulative effects, but hereditary interference in development spells mental retardation when the normal genetic endowment is distributed by abnormal genes or abnormal numbers of chromosomes.

Intelligence tests provide an estimate of an individual's capacity for convergent thought. It is the ability to arrive at the correct solution to a problem on the basis of the given information. Such tests do not provide a measure of the ability to reorganize given information into various forms of divergent thinking. Little progress will be made in understanding creativity without standardized tests of the capacity for divergent thought. Creative thinking is significant in cognitive functioning, but its measures are not correlated with I.Q. tests; indeed, adolescents with high I.Q. scores do no better on creativity tasks than patients with low I.Q. scores. Intelligence tests only yield information about relative brightness without inferences about how people think or about their development of intellectual functioning or about the manner of solving problems.

The limitations of concrete operational thought from seven to eleven are overcome at puberty with formal operational thought, a radical shift in the way adolescents think. This is propositional, for the adolescent can formulate statements about possible relations in the world and then operate on those the way he was able to operate on objects and events in previous concrete operations. He is no longer limited to what is perceptually present, for he is able to think in terms of the possible and to realize the abstract nature of his propositions. Propositional thinking gradually becomes more general and more organized. Thought not restricted to the concrete embodies more abstract conceptual attainments, manifested by the adolescent's concepts of the intangibles that bind human relationships—love, justice, equality, charity, society, infinity.

The mental age according to the I.Q. is an index of maturation of the mind increasing at a rate determined by intrinsic and environmental factors. Effective teaching and stimulating experiences sharpen the wits and accelerate mental capacity; otherwise, the mentality may lag behind. The fallacy that mental age proceeds at a steady rate independent of surroundings and ultimately attains a maximum level controlled only by intrinsic factors led to erroneous sorting of students. It is still difficult to determine when mental development reaches maturity—somewhere between fifteen and twenty-five years of age. Intellectual performance continues to improve through knowledge, training and experience even though the mental capacity to deal with intellectual material does not increase but the know-what and know-how enable it to function more smoothly. Most university students admitted on merit have I.Q.s of 120 or over, while most noneducable youths have I.Q.s of 60 or less. Minds differ still more than faces.

The nature of general intelligence measured by I.Q. tests depends on the particular ensemble of items, hence it becomes necessary to measure different abilities depending on the need for prediction or diagnosis. Thurstone considers six abilities involving operational contents and products: verbal, numerical, spatial, reasoning and memory abilities. The first verbal ability is vocabulary size, which depends on recognition of words, measured by multiple choice vocabulary tests. The second verbal ability is word fluency, which deals with active recall of words to fit a given demand. Numerical ability involves facility in arithmetic measured by problems that can be solved correctly in a given time limit. Spatial ability, two- or three-dimensional, provides better measures of the ability to think abstractly or to form general concepts than do verbal tests. Reasoning ability is independent of number, spatial and verbal abilities and comes closest to what is usually considered to be intelligence, yet current reasoning tests have considerable verbal or spatial components which do not correlate highly. Memory is distinct from the other five abilities but may not be unitary in the same sense as the others because there are different mechanisms for short-term and long-term storage as well as separate memory abilities for different types of material. Measurement of memory does not test a skill acquired in the past because the adolescent learns something while taking the test. Motivation thus assumes a more important role than in the measurement of other abilities.

The concept of separate abilities is based on factor analyses of batteries of tests which group themselves according to common abilities. The primary nature of specific abilities lends itself for application in the differentiation or prediction of success in various curricula and jobs, in the stability of the factor over different age ranges, in the cross-cultural generalities of the ability patterns, in the comparability of different ability levels, in the different effects of mental illness, in the evaluation of different rates of development. Human abilities with specific genes acquired during evolution need special conditions to come to fruition in particular individuals. A minimum of social interaction is necessary for normal development. Differences in the amount of stimulation lead to differences in brain chemistry that mediate differences in ability; conversely, lack of mental stimulation has an adverse effect on mental development.

The major source of differences in abilities is no longer considered the quality of schooling but rather the preschool experiences plus innate differences. Skeels transferred a child from an orphanage to an institution for mentally retarded who showed considerable I.Q. increase compared with those who remained in the orphanage because of the social stimulation in the mental institution as compared with isolation in the orphanage. Early home environment is more critical than later periods of childhood; but we do not know if the stimulation does as much good as restraint and deprivation do harm. Mankind has not changed drastically over the past half million years, except for the vast improvement in technical skills, but the increase in man's technological ability has not been equally increased in moral and spiritual development evolving in mental maturation.

Academic Achievement

The g factor continues to be manifest in adolescent behavior as general adaptability in stimulation situations. The g factor becomes much more evident than ever before in exercising special mental abilities. The increasing mental growth requires appropriate environmental situations to bring those abilities to the fore. There is no sudden spurt of mental development at the onset of puberty for either boys or girls. Specific mental functions evolve as a continuum of growth and development from infancy and culminate at maturity. The ability to concentrate upon a situation or to continue a task is ever individual. If the attention span is short, the interest slips from one to another. An adolescent gradually gains the ability to concentrate on the task at hand, but personal interest in the activity is a determining factor in his willingness to concentrate effectively. Environmental conditions always interfere with concentration. The ideal setting for study is an isolated room but the adolescent exposed to conversation, radio, television and telephone adapts to the circumstances and resorts to differential hearing in order to concentrate upon his studies.

The ability to memorize is determined by the intensity and duration of a stimulus and the personal feelings attached to it.

Pleasant experiences are remembered longer than annoyances, but embarrassing situations arising from social immaturity may so affect the adolescent's self-regard that he becomes emotionally involved at the time of its occurrence. More serious is the fact that he remembers it for a long time unless he redeems himself by displaying social ease or, until he recognizes the relative unimportance of the incident. Adolescent memory may be rote or logical. Youth finds verbatim memorization monotonous and prefers to recall meaningful ideas presented in his own words. Rote memory is effective if youth understands the meaning of what he is memorizing, has a personal interest in the material to be memorized, and gets the commendation he expects to receive for his performance.

Imagination derives from inherited potentials and/or environmental stimulations. It may be the determining factor in special aptitudes which are transformed by training into superperformance, i.e. music, art, mathematics, writing or other specific abilities. Prognostic tests may reveal an adolescent's special aptitudes but the possession of such specific abilities is not productive of full realization unless motivated by intensive participation in appropriate learning experiences. Adolescents give their imagination free rein, expressing their imaginary dreams in poems or idealistic stories which reveal their developing philosophy of life or personal ambitions. Youth expresses the mood of the moment or the play of imagination with total disregard of technical accuracy of the performance. But youth can be encouraged to develop realistically controlled imagination; the interested teacher recognizes the caliber of imagination and encourages cultivation of special training of aptitudes.

Problem solving is based on imagination and reasoning. The degree of skill attained depends on the upper limits of mental development. Every adolescent has a specific ability to think and judge correctly, develop insight about people, objects and situations, ever enhanced by training. He usually depends upon creative imagination or paraphrased published opinions or garnered conversations of adults without any original thinking of his own. Reasoning can only be valid if it represents the mental maturation and experimental evaluation of the maturing individual. An adolescent can thus be gradually helped to achieve control of his imagination through better approaches to the realities of life and be inducted gradually into problem-solving situations.

Productive thinking is sparked by intense awareness of a difficulty. A suggested solution springs into mind, is accepted or rejected, and new combinations of thoughts arise from rational association, from cerebral fancy or chance circumstance. The fertile mind tries a large number and a variety of combinations. The sound thinker withholds judgment and remains in doubt when the evidence is insufficient. Imagination rarely gives one a correct answer, for most ideas have to be discarded, but curiosity comes to the fore unless allowed to atrophy after childhood. Once youth contemplates approaches to his problems, the mind tends to follow the same line of thought each time, profitable and unprofitable. The only way to free the thoughts from such conditioning is to abandon the problem temporarily and to discuss it with peers, parents and teachers.

Learning is a modification of behavior by experience from intrauterine stimulation through life's vicissitudes. The ability to learn is partly inborn, the intelligent learning quickly and the subnormal slowly, with no qualitative difference in factual content. Conditioned learning is either Pavlovian or Skinnerian; the one based on the classical experimental dog which salivates when presented with food regularly, just as verbal presentation of a favored menu will cause the mouth to water; and the other on conditioning of the trial and error kind with an internal reward for the correct response and punishment for the incorrect. Insight learning is characterized by sudden improvement in the task learned due to inner neural reorganization of the task. Good teaching facilitates insight learning by emphasizing those factors that allow the student to see wholes rather than parts or by understanding rather than by rote. Social learning takes into one's own personality the behavior of significant human figures around the individual. Such identification offers many ways of learning to cope with the environment modified by one's own experience.

Memory comprises the storage and retrieval of information. We have a genetic DNA memory, an immunological memory, a psychic memory, and many other memories in life processes. In particular, the psychic memory embodies learning and remembering, corresponding to storage and retrieval of information. There are two varieties of psychic memory. One is the brief memory for seconds or minutes, such as the ability to repeat the sequence of numbers that have been read out and lost beyond all recall, subserved by a spatiotemporal pattern of propagation impulse in a reverberating circulation. Retrieval is possible as long as this specific pattern is preserved to form a dynamic engram. The second is distinguished by its enduring characteristic needed for a lifetime and survives even when the CNS is reduced to a quiescent state in deep anesthesia or in coma. Such long-term memory is built into the fine CNS architecture as memory traces with synaptic structural changes. The structural basis of memory is delineated by a specific reorganization of neuron associations with the engram in a vast square of neurons widely spread over the cerebral cortex and the subcortical ganglia.

The activity of millions of neurons partakes in the recall of any memory; it does not belong exclusively to any one engram, for each neuron and each synaptic junction is built into many engrams. Thinking is the mental manipulation of information that has been learned at a relatively simple level or at the highest degree of abstraction. Intelligence is determined by inborn factors susceptible to environmental modification but pure intelligence has a genetically determined ceiling beyond which none of us can go. Applied intelligence reflected by I.Q. consists of that part of our genetic endowment we actually use and is affected by emotional and social forces. Most tests measure a limited number of group factors, especially a verbal factor, numerical factor, spatial factor and mechanical factor.

Academic achievement is the resultant of speed or the ability to solve problems quickly and of the power or ceiling of an individual's production regardless of the time spent. An adolescent's cognitive style is remarkably consistent and recognizable while he is thinking, learning, memorizing or perceiving. Creativity depends not merely on the ability to solve problems but on the ability to invent. Many creative individuals are not especially intelligent in the sense that they can score high I.Q. tests, while many individuals who score high on I.Q. tests may be quite uncreative. Apparently, a convergent type of person performs well in normal I.Q. tests in which an answer has to be reasoned out from a number of alternatives. The divergent type does better on I.Q. tests in which the problems are couched in an open-ended manner when the answer has to be invented. What chemical changes in neurons are involved in the storage of information? RNA of the neurons is markedly increased, accompanied by accelerated protein synthesis as memory traces when the memories conduct impulses. DNA in the nucleus of egg and sperm is the information code of the gene which informs each oncoming generation how to make a person. It synthesizes RNA as a template which produces the cell's proteins and enzymes.

Intellectual potential arises genetically while capability emerges only to the extent to which maturation forces and environmental opportunities promote its development and expression. Capability represents a degree of actual functional attainment while potential attainment lies in the future. Capability is subject to observation, examination and elevation while potentiality is concealed power which cannot be observed clinically though predictable to some extent. Biological individuality is responsible for the variability of endowed potentialities in every individual. The variability in environmental opportunities, even among siblings, further leads to a wide range of capability levels extending from superior through average, below average, shading through ill-defined variables into minimal subnormal, while poor genetic potential or harmful environment further lowers the range of capabilities.

Man is not realizing his full potential despite remarkable capabilities. He needs marked improvement in obvious imperfections as a psychosocial being. He can be upgraded, for his genetic potential far exceeds his normal visible expression. Anatomical development needs thousands of years but social development can emerge in decades. Actually, man at best is using his brain at about one-tenth of its full capacity. Every individual tends to improve his best capabilities and to understand and control his worst. He cannot be changed in genetics which takes eons of time but he can be changed by psychological means. Psychochemicals can increase verbal capability in some individuals, competence in mathematical and artistic capabilities in others. If youth were to force his brain to work at only half the real capacity, he would be able to learn forty languages, memorize the encyclopedia, and complete the required college courses in a year.

The gap between potential and capability may be considerable. Human potentials are established at conception through the transmission of the genetic code in the parental germ cells. Individual variations are reflected in the ultimate capabilities of the organism. If the genetic code is transmitted with some defect, the potential of the organism is impaired. The chromosomal defect may involve the whole organism, as in Down's disease, or in enzyme abnormalities, as in phenylketonuria. Whatever the degree of genetic impairment, there is neurological disorganization in the individual. Adverse environmental forces may impede or distort neurological organization with normal or abnormal potential. The potential of the normal organism is neither observable nor measurable. The potential of the individual who is neurologically disorganized is even more of an enigma. Whatever potential exists in the neurologically disorganized child, it must reside in the functionally depressed or underdeveloped cerebral tissues which might be raised to effective levels of action. The therapeutic means must be the same basic physiological developmental process that would have advanced the child's capabilities if he had not remained immature.

Psychologic Deterrents

There are almost no limits to the discoveries of how the adolescent brain operates—in health and illness, in work and play, in school and home, in waking and in sleep, in day- and night-dreaming, in calm and under tension. The question is how far we can apply these discoveries for brain power as well as for clinical cure. Intelligence develops at the mercy of the psychological environment. It can be increased to some extent but is invariably diminished by emotional disturbances, the underlying basis for emotional immaturity in the intelligent youth who makes great demands on life for opportunities to use his ability. To the dull mind all nature is leaden; to the illumined mind the whole world sparkles. An adolescent who differs significantly from his peers is apt to find difficulties along the road. Sometimes, the superior youth elaborates his difficulties until they come close to being a psychological problem, although actual psychosis in the highly intellectual is not more significant than in the normal intelligent adolescent. The direct speech of feeling is allegorical and cannot be replaced by anything, hence youth remains a block-head, more ready to feel and digest than to think and consider. The test of a first-rate intelligence is the ability to hold two opposed ideas in the mind at the same time and still retain the ability to function.

The mentally superior adolescent has severe personality and emotional struggles in childhood as a result of failure to fit in with children of the same chronological age. A superior intelligence in youth is a mixed blessing, carrying with it the possibility of the highest leadership and accomplishments, on the one hand, and the greatest loneliness and misunderstanding, on the other. An infinite variety of opposing influences stand between intellectual ability and its full utilization. First and foremost, the adolescent must have some urge to use its intellectual ability. The possession of abilities in themselves constitutes a powerful urge, and the intelligent adolescent constantly seeks ways of applying his abilities in the choice of a vocation, but mental difficulties may arise from thwarting his mentality. Intelligence in chains loses in lucidity what it gains in intensity.

The intellectually superior adolescent is conscious of differing from his fellows and is often regarded by them with suspicion. He is apt to become asocial and often antisocial and thus develop emotional problems which prevent full expression of his intellectual abilities. Emotional maladaptation is not a necessary concomitant of superior intellectual capacities, for many superior adolescents are able to use effectively the abilities they possess. Neither is a superior intellect a necessary drawback to prowess in other social fields such as athletics. Nevertheless, the use of superior intellectual endowment has more exacting requirements in life than that of the less gifted. Clinically, the possession of intelligence carries with it the need for furnishing that intellect with adequate raw materials with which to work to avoid maladjustments. What hunger is in relation to food, zest is in relation to life for the bright youth. He soon realizes that pleasures of the senses are temporary, that pleasures of the heart lead to sorrow, and pleasures of the mind to eternal bliss.

Intelligent adolescents seek out friends whose intelligence matches their own or is just slightly inferior to it. The process depends partly upon the screening out of those of lesser intelligence by the schooling process. If economic and other factors are equal, the average intelligence of a group of adolescents whose entire schooling consisted of grade school will be lower than that of a corresponding group with a high school education. Similarly, higher intellectual levels are found in college graduates. The fact that these averages may be placed in a row according to schooling is no guarantee that such a generality would extend to a college graduate or to an illiterate, for other factors determine how much schooling an individual gets.

The intelligent young woman is often limited by the very possession of high intelligence, for it must be used in one way or another and cannot be hidden easily. The myth of the superior male is so strong throughout the Anglo-Saxon society that few young men will marry or associate for a long time with a young woman who can surpass his intelligence. That limits the field of selection to men who are equal or superior and diminishes very rapidly with each slight increase in intellectual level. Clearly, the intellectually superior adolescent suffers emotionally because of social difficulties which follow upon his or her differences from the accepted norm. The choice of work, hobbies, interests and adolescent mates depends to a large extent on intellectual capacities.

Athletic pastimes have their appeal at any intellectual level yet some sedentary hobbies are more selective in their appeal. Contract bridge requires greater intelligence than gin rummy, while amateur mathematics would not be considered entertaining by one whose intellectual capacities are satisfied by crossword puzzles. Frequently the type of hobbies chosen may be a very good index of the intellectual characteristics of an adolescent. No youth is really happy or safe without a hobby and it makes precious little difference what the outside interests may be—botany, flowers, gardening, fishing, mountaineering—anything will do so long as he straddles a hobby and rides it hard. The number of hobbies a youth has may likewise point out his intellectual status. In fact, the drive to use intellectual ability intensively or extensively is one of the chief clinical features of the superior adolescent. In the search he becomes a true snob that never rests; there is always a higher goal to attain, and there are, by the same token, always more and more people to look down upon.

Abstract Thinking

Profundity of thought belongs to youth; clarity to the mature. Adolescent thinking is the endeavor to capture reality by ideas. The brightest flashes in the world of thought are incomplete until they have been proved to have their counterparts in the world of reality. Thinking is hard work for you can't bear burdens and ideas at the same time. But common sense is as rare as genius even though it emerges in the mental maturation of the pre-puberal child. The material world at last begins to make sense to him with the categories, positions and relationships of objects in space and time. But the child must have concrete objects before him to be able to deal with them coherently. It is not until adolescence that abstract thought enables youth to reason about events as well as with events themselves. A fine logical apparatus can now deal with hypothetical ideas as well as with actuality. But the brain is not completely formed until sexuality has come into bloom. Reason becomes youth's faculty for grasping the world by thought, while intelligence enables him to manipulate the world with the help of thought.

The encounter with the self extends to the intellectual development which takes a new surge between ages eleven and fifteen with the introduction of propositional logic. The mode of thinking shifts from the concrete to the hypothetical deductive level. The older child reasons about existing objects to establish relations between them. The world of abstract relations superimposes itself on the world of factual situations. But the structural perfection of thought is achieved by age fifteen when formal thinking is applied to everything, for all things become a matter of logical structuring. This intellectual development gives the adolescent his proper character. He reasons about the least topical of subjects remote from his personal experience, in scientific, philosophical, artistic, political and social problems. The adolescent plays games with ideas despite lack of experience, sense of relativity and self-criticism. He discovers himself in these discussions, encounters himself while detaching some factual reasoning. He develops a sense of originality and of responsibility, ever engaged by his own liberty. The intellectual poses questions subtly preoccupied with self-awareness. He is ever occupied with himself, complains of his looks but not of his brains. All his mind's activity is easy if it is not subjected to reality.

The sudden surge of abstract intellectual development of youth produces diffuse emotional effects that explain his unique life style. He reveals a special intensity or volatility of feeling with rapid fluctuation of object choice. He goes out of his way to find emotional experiences, seeks frequent immediate gratification for pleasure and so prefers rock music to Mozart. He has to be kept constantly interested for he cannot tolerate anxiety, appears unaware of the consequences of his actions and misunderstands the feelings of others. He lacks the knack of self-criticism, the ability to perceive contradiction, the incongruity and absurdity in himself and his behavior. He cannot concern himself with persons, objects and events that do not impinge upon him personally. He gradually envisions people as having ways of life of their own without relevance to him at the core of the world.

The adolescent is plagued into ambivalence and uncertainty. The old assurances of childhood wane with a degree of nostalgia but the templates of the new are alarming. All certainties are questioned, ever asking what am I? What do I want? What is my value? Am I up to standard? He does not understand himself and feels not understood. He senses himself and withdraws further into himself. He knows not what behavior to adopt and, indeed, refuses to behave. He talks back loudly, arrogantly and aggressively but he seeks to evaluate himself by his skills, his eccentricities and his convictions. He detaches himself from all that reminds him of his former role to affirm his new status. He liberates himself from his parents with guilt feelings and regressions. Adults have poor tolerance for loss of prestige and respond by irony and coercion that aggravates the adolescent's rebelliousness. Youth shrewdly judges adults without consideration, exposing their hypocrisy against his sincerity. The conflict of the generations is not complete, for many an adult's behavior strikes an harmonious cord in the adolescent's conscience. It enables a form of limitation and identification with values that are of primary importance to him. He designs his permanent ideal through real or fantasy personalities representing diverse categories of human beings.

The adolescent likes to record his discoveries in an intimate diary of first facts and events. He quotes from his readings, encounters, records, impressions, reflections and confessions and attempts self-analysis. He finds security and rivalry amongst his peers, insures his security by strict conformance to the group with total mimicry in contrast to the emancipation from the family situation. He becomes a perfect snob, adapting new customs and fashions; gives himself value and distinguishes himself from his equals by bragging, by exploits and by opinions. But he usually meets an alter ego in his group, a favorite friend with whom he searches to explore himself. The two help each other to become aware of themselves in the course of joint adventures, experiences and confidential conversations. These friendships have a narcissistic component of passionate character. He finally discovers someone who understands him and takes him seriously and respects him.

Juvenile friendships constitute a rehearsal for love in the presence of witnesses. They confirm his personality and identity which contribute to the fixation of his traits and orientation of positive tasks of existence. The experience with a friend of his own sex enables him to face a friend of the opposite sex. Exploratory activities on both sides commence first figuratively and then literally with flirtations and intimacies. The adolescent is a ward of his life aimed at a future while the child lives in the present like an adult attached to his daily tasks. He detaches himself from the present and dreams of the future in exaggerated form. He projects plans created by his abstract mental structure; but being squeezed between child and adulthood, i.e. treated as a child at one time and as an adult another, creates delay and respite. He always waits for something to happen—awaits a revelation amidst his yearnings. He lives a fluctuant existence of extremes, exploring his life in every way despite uncertainties, confronted abruptly by a world entirely different from that to which he is accustomed.

Mental Growth

Intellectual growth emerges from active responses by the developing child. The mind is like a plant, appropriating and assimilating that about him which responds to that which is within him. Information derived from his environment becomes formative instead of informative when both body and mind respond creatively to the impact-yielding "schemas." The assimilation of new experiences increases their complexity to enable achievement of more complex accommodations. Even if environmental stimulation wanes, meanings become reorganized in the mind in consonance with other meanings. The child's response to environmental stimuli is manifest in the structural development of the nervous system. The brain develops with use and wastes with disuse throughout life. It is ever preparing itself for particular events at critical periods to enable new accomplishments. Each area of the brain shows immense variations in the state of development for the child progresses as various parts of the brain mature and come into active service.

The child does not learn to walk or talk until his brain is ready according to the individual timetable. The powers of speech are closely synchronized with the developmental tempo. If the child is immersed in a sea of language, he passes from one level of comprehension to the next. If deafness or other disorder delays language acquisition, or if brain injuries in early life destroy language already acquired, he can still make favorable progress up to age of ten years. A child up to ten can learn foreign languages the natural way, but in the early teens, as the brain finally matures, it switches off its powers of spontaneous language acquisition. The slowly maturing frontal lobes are required for correct responses to verbal instructions, hence damage to the frontal lobes leads to abnormal performance in adolescents. The immaturity of the brain makes it physically impossible to do what such youth is told to do. He understands the requests but his brain is unable to act on them. It is imperative for parents and teachers to realize the nature of the immaturity in order to cope effectively at every turn in the everyday life of the affected child. Once their understanding is clear, adolescent interrelationship with adults is made easier.

The child perceives the adult as omnipotent and believes in omnipotent justice. As he learns to play cooperatively with other children he makes rules of logic that gradually give way to propositional reasoning at puberty. Rigid equality leads to a sense of equity. The child of eleven begins to think in terms of possibilities, considering reality no longer as that part of the possible which might occur, but that which has actually occurred. He can now hold some variables constant while manipulating others, but it is not until fifteen that he can hold a number of variables constant and vary one variable at a time, a capacity that lays the foundation for the ultimate involvement of the scientific method of thinking.

The adolescent can view the world, its morality, and value systems from the standpoint of the possibles—from a "what would happen if" position. He not only builds new theories or rehabilitates old ones but develops a concept of life to enable him to assert himself and create something applicable to him individually. This initiates the formation of a philosophy of life based on his past, present and future that will pave the way for a greater personal success than his predecessors. The formal thought of the adolescent is the key to understanding his mental processes. The little-minded adolescent's thoughts move in such small circles that five minutes' evaluation gives you an arc long enough to determine the whole curve. But an arc in the movement of a large intellect does not sensibly differ from a straight line.

Intellectual capacity expands rapidly during adolescence with the growing ability to handle abstract concepts and new ways of conceptualizing time and space and one's relationship to it. Indeed, the intellect cuts loose from the concrete events of daily life and becomes a powerful force for better or worse in the regulation of daily behavior. It is a process of extension of rationality at its best and a flight into unreality at its worst. The adolescent vacillates between romantic, highly intellectualized theory building and impulsive everyday behavior which bears little relationship to his high ideals, principles and theories. As he imagines the world as it might be, he develops resentment of the world as it is. His ability to dream of a radically different future enables him to build a world of the imagination that serves as an ideal model and as an escape from the trials of the present turmoil.

Freedom of thought constitutes man's primary instrument of survival. The inherent drive to use the mind is so great that suppression of independent thinking has never been complete. The freedom that matters is the freedom to know, freedom of opinion, of discussion and of action. Such a freedom does not limit the freedom of others. On the contrary, the realization of the spiritual freedom of individuals will make of justice and friendship the true foundations of social life. Youth must have the freedom to make by their own efforts the utmost of their lives to develop themselves as persons, to give their talents full scope, to live according to their ideals, to control their destiny. This is the freedom of fulfillment.

Youthful heretics have always risen to challenge aged orthodoxies. The human race owes most of its valuable progress to adolescent heretics who insist on changing behavior patterns to fit tested new experience and knowledge, independent of the ancestral or authoritarian dictates. Uncritical acceptance of parental or local patterns of thinking may be considered good, but world opinion now differs openly. We owe almost all our knowledge to those who have differed. Youth's goal is a society which gives each individual optimum conditions for leading a full and responsible life with the full development of his talents rather than a society for the maximum production of wealth, or for the maximum development of trade or for the maximum concentration of power in a governing oligarchy with maximum subservience and passive obedience of the people. Youth always dissents with perpetual intoxication from a fever of the mind.

Early adolescence reveals marked restlessness and argumentativeness, while late adolescence reveals tranquility with some interest in adult affairs as a result of the development of abstract thinking. The ability to reason permits the adolescent to explore possible actions and judge the value of each plan before selecting the one to carry out. Reason gives harmony to irrational impulses and makes truth prevail. The older adolescent has the ability to evaluate the course of action and effective goals instead of proceeding impulsively until blocked. He becomes more and more involved with adult society and thrives on idealistic endeavors. He may even alter his appearance to conform to the requisites of a suitable vocation.

A professional role may be rejected because lengthy pursuit of knowledge and training is not worth the eventual reward. Some adolescents are content with a limited socioeconomic level rather than pursue far-flung sacrifices into the future. Others reject adult society as a whole because nonconformists repudiate world values and even plot to destroy the entire basis of society. Actually, both conformists and nonconformists play the same game except that the former decides that he could succeed in the adult world by accepting the rules of the game while the latter simply wants no part of it. Both groups choose a course of action by seeking an identity and relate it to idealism. Commitment to an ideal may take precedence over every other aspect of life because it provides a motive for living and fills a childhood void.

Adolescents are what their mothers made them, for their caliber is determined more by mothers than by fathers. But character cannot be acquired at ease; only through experience of trial and suffering can the soul be strengthened, the mind sharpened, the vision cleared, the ambition inspired and achievement fulfilled. Happiness is not the end of life, character is; it begins to form at the first pinch of anxiety about an individual. When youth lacks character, he is badly in need of a new way of life. Adolescent idealism and energy alter basic social and cultural forces to bring about revolutionary changes. Idealism springs from deep feelings but feelings are nothing without the formulated idea that keeps them whole. They constitute an imaginative understanding of that which is desirable in that which is possible. In due time, in spite of endless adolescence, they usually accept adult prerogatives but resent adult influence. There are always conflicts in the desires, expectations and social changes sought by late adolescents with those of adults who want to preserve the social structure to which they are accustomed. The mental caliber of the adolescent should be judged by the way he sees himself, by the quality of his values, by the formulation of his goals, by the state of his sexual development, by his concern for others, by his awareness of his preparation for a vocation, and by the successful separation from his parents, the assumption of self-responsibility and the achievement of an identity as an independent individual.

REFERENCES

Abercrombie, M. L. J.: *The Anatomy of Judgment*. London, Hutchison, 1960.
Achenback, T. *et al.*: Cue-learning and problem-learning strategies in normal and retarded children. *Child Develop.*, 39:827, 1968.
Bayley, N.: Behavioral correlates of mental growth. *Am. Psychol.*, 23:1-17, 1968.
Bernstein, N. R.: *Diminished People*. Boston, Little, Brown, 1970.

Bettelheim, B.: *The Empty Fortress.* Canada, Collier-Macmillan, 1967.

Bijou, S. W.: Research on the academic education of the retarded. In G. A. Jervis (Ed.): *Expanding Concepts in Mental Retardation.* Springfield, Charles C Thomas, 1968.

Bindra, D.: *Motivation: A Systematic Reinterpretation.* New York, Ronald, 1959.

Birch, H. G. (Ed.): *Brain Damage in Children.* New York, Williams and Wilkins, 1964.

Blatt, B. *et al.:* Dissonant notions concerning disordered children and their educability. *J. Educ. Ment. Retard., 1:11,* 1966.

Bloomberg, M.: An inquiry into the relationship between field independence-dependence and creativity. *J. Psychol., 67:127-40,* 1967.

Brower, D.: Academic underachievement. *J. Psychol., 66:299-302,* 1967.

Bruner, J. S.: The growth of the mind. *Am. Psychol. Assoc., 9:4,* 1965.

Budner, S. *et al.:* The minority retardate. *Soc. Serv. Rev., 43:174,* 1969.

Carter, D. B. (Ed.): *Interdisciplinary Approaches to Learning Disorders.* Philadelphia, Chilton, 1970.

Chess, S. *et al.: Temperament and Behavior Disorders in Children.* New York, NYU Press, 1968.

Clarke, A. M. *et al.* (Eds.): *Mental Deficiency: The Changing Outlook.* New York, Free Press, 1965.

Clausen, J.: Assessment of behavior characteristics in mental retardates. *Proc. Am. Psychopathol. Assoc. 56:2708,* 1967.

Dexter, L. A.: *The Tyranny of Schooling: An Inquiry into the Problems of Stupidity.* New York, Basic Books, 1964.

Di Cara, L. V.: Learning in the automatic nervous system. *Sci. Am. 222:30-19,* 1970.

Earl, G. J. *et al.: Subnormal Personalities.* London, Bailliere, Tindall & Cox, 1961.

Eastham, R. D. *et al.: Clinical Pathology in Mental Retardation.* Bristol, John Wright, 1968.

Eccles, J. C.: *Facing Reality.* New York, Springer-Verlag, 1970.

Elkin, F. *et al.:* The myth of adolescent culture. *Ann. Am. Acad. Polit. Soc. Sci.,* 1944.

Erikson, E. H.: *Insight and Responsibility.* New York, Norton, 1964.

Finger, J. A. *et al.:* Non-intellective predictors of academic success in school and college. *Sch. Rev., 73:14-29,* 1965.

Freeman, R. D.: Drug effects on learning in children. *J. Special Educ., 1:17,* 1966.

Freud, A.: *Normality and Pathology in Childhood.* New York, International Universities Press, 1965.

Frierson, E. C. *et al.: Educating Children with Learning Disabilities.* New York, Appleton-Century-Crofts, 1967.

Gartner, M.: *Mental Handicap, Aspects of Curative Education.* Aberdeen University Press, 1966.

Gofman, H.: Etiologic factors in learning disorders of children. *J. Neurol. Sci.* 2:262-70, 1965.

Hammar, S. L.: School underachievement in the adolescent. *Pediatrics, 40:* 373-381, 1967.

Harris, B. R. *et al.:* Intelligence, personality, and achievement. *Can. Psychiatr. Assoc. J., 13:*335-9, 1968.

Hunt, J. McV.: *Intelligence and Experience.* New York, Ronald, 1961.

Inhelder, B. *et al.: The Growth of Logical Thinking from Childhood to Adolescence.* New York, Basic Books, 1958.

Jacobs, P. A. *et al.:* Aggressive behavior, mental subnormality and the XYZ male. *Nature, 208:*1351-1352, 1965.

Jahoda, M.: *Current Concepts of Positive Mental Health.* New York, Basic Books, 1958.

Jensen, A. R.: How much can we boost I.Q. and scholastic achievement? *Harvard Educ. Rev., 39:*1, 1969.

Justak, J. F.: Intelligence tests and personality structure. *Proc. Am. Psychopath Assoc., 56:*282-97, 1967.

Kaplan, B. (Ed.): *Studying Personality Cross-culturally.* Evanston, Row Peterson, 1961.

Klineberg, S. L.: Changes in outlook on the future between childhood and adolescence. *J. Pers. Soc. Psychol., 7:*185-93, 1967.

Kohut, S. A.: The abnormal child: his impact on the family. *Phys. Ther., 46:* 160, 1966.

Kugelmass, I. N.: *The Autistic Child.* Springfield, Charles C Thomas, 1970.

Luria, A. R. *et al.: Speech and Development of Mental Processes in the Child.* London, Staples, 1966.

Martin, W. A.: Word-fluency intellect or personality? *J. Genet. Psychol., 118:*17-24, 1971.

Mead, M. *et al.: Childhood in Contemporary Cultures.* Chicago, University of Chicago, 1955.

Merenda, F. F. *et al.:* Cross-cultural perceptions of the ideal self-concept. *Int. Rev. Appl. Psychol., 18:*129, 1969.

Mowrer, O. H.: *Learning Theory and Behavior.* New York, Wiley, 1960.

Neimark, E. D. *et al.:* The development of logical problem solving strategies. *Child Dev., 38:*107-117, 1967.

Olshansky, S.: Parents' response to a mentally defective child. *Ment. Retard., 4:*21, 1966.

Pang, H. *et al.:* Personality traits and handwriting characteristics. *Percept. Motor Skills, 26:*1082, 1968.

Piaget, J.: The intellectual development of the adolescent. In G. Caplan and S. Lebovici (Eds.): *Adolescence: Psychosocial Perspectives.* New York, Basic Books, 1969, pp. 22-26.

Pinneau, S. R. *et al.*: Development of mental abilities. *Rev. Educ. Res., 28:* 392-400, 1958.

Posner, C. M.: *Mental Retardation: Diagnosis and Treatment.* New York, Harper & Row, 1969.

Raben, M. S.: Growth hormone. *N. Engl. J. Med., 266:*31, 82, 1962.

Ratcliffe, A.: *The Child and Reality.* London, George Allen & Unwin, 1970.

Reisman, F.: *The Culturally Deprived Child.* New York, Harper, 1962.

Rubins, J. L.: The problem of the acute identity crisis in adolescence. *Am. J. Psychoanal., 28:*37-47, 1968.

Schwalb, E.: Clinical considerations of cerebral dysfunction in children. *N. Y. State J. Med., 67:*2320-2324, 1967.

Segal, S. S.: *No Child Is Ineducable.* New York, Pergamon, 1967.

Sternlicht, M.: Psychotherapeutic techniques useful with the mentally retarded. *Psychiatr. Qu., 39:*84, 1965.

Szurek, S. A. *et al.*: Mental retardation and psychotherapy. In I. Philips (Ed.): *Prevention and Treatment of Mental Retardation.* New York, Basic Books, 1966.

Tansley, A. E. *et al.*: *The Education of Slow Learning Children.* London, Routledge and Kegan Paul, 1965.

Vernon, P. E.: *The Measurement of Abilities.* London, University London Press, 1956; *Intelligence and Attainment Tests.* London, University London Press, 1960.

Walter, W. G.: *The Living Brain.* London, Penguin Books, 1961.

Watzlawick, P. *et al.*: *Pragmatics of Human Communication.* New York, Norton, 1967.

Weihs, T. J.: Differential diagnosis of backward children. In Pietzner (Ed.): *Aspects of Curative Education.* Aberdeen University Press, 1966.

Williams, I. A.: Management of the adolescent with cerebral palsy. *Lancet,* p. 1126, 1969.

Williams, M.: *Mental Testing in Clinical Practice.* New York, Pergamon, 1965.

Winter, S. K. *et al.*: Capacity for self-direction. *J. Consult. Clin. Psychol., 32:*25-41, 1968.

Wolstenholme and Porter (Eds.): *Mongolism.* Ciba Foundation, No. 25. Churchill, 1967.

Zimmerman, K. A.: How adolescents view themselves. *Med. Arts Sci., 22:* 49-56, 1968.

CHAPTER IV

EMOTIONAL IMMATURITY

There is a side to human behavior in everyday life
which is not a thing of intellect,
which is irrational and emotional but important.
It is the main spring of most of what we do
and a great deal of what we feel.

L ife is the enjoyment of emotion derived from the past and
aimed at the future. It is being explored by scientists but
neglected by physicians. Both realize that there is nothing more
injurious to the character and to the intellect of youth than the
suppression of generous emotion. It engages all major regions
of the brain rather than independent centers and must have a
high degree of maturity to be effective for the adolescent experience. How shall one who is so weak in childhood become really
strong during adolescence? We only change our fancies but
they must be mature fancies. The emotional mind changes one's
countenance unexpectedly for good or for evil and lifts one up,
if adequate and balanced, or distorts one side of the being, if
inadequate or unbalanced. Emotional maturity involves a realistic
concept of ego identity as its foundation that creates not only
the capacity for functioning agreeably but also the ability to
enjoy it all fully, while emotional immaturity warps the style of
adolescent life with deficiencies which must be detected and
corrected before lifelong patterns become established irreversibly.

Lack of a Sense of Reality

The world of theatre is not life in miniature but life enormously
magnified, life hideously exaggerated. The external world is
viewed by the adolescent as a distant stage on which skillful players are easily producing a successful performance. The young
spectator can hardly imagine that he will ever have sufficient skill
to handle anything more than a walk-on part. At other times,
he sees the world as a cast of untutored players to be molded

116

to his sense of drama. He shifts from seeing the reality as a malleable medium in which he can implant an image of his inner struggles to viewing it as a relatively fixed situation to which he must mold himself. The younger adolescent views himself as the undiscovered director while the older adolescent gradually accepts a less inflated role in the production of life.

Ego function controls three worlds of reality—the world of external reality, the world of imagination, and the world of linguistic expression. We see only what we look for, and we look for only what we know. Boys see the objective world differently from the way girls see it; a man's world is different from a woman's world; and every individual's world looks different from the other's due to congenital differences in perceptual, CNS and motor equipment, and to acquired experiences. The world of imagination never becomes completely realistic of reality, but always warmer, more colorful and more vivid. Imagination can serve creative and recreational purposes; it can transcend space and time, change monotony into adventure, picture escape when doomed, daydream of the future. For youth, it remains a refuge from the world of facts, a world into which he can withdraw when objective reality becomes drab. The verbal world presents a comprehensive symbolic framework embracing many aspects of reality, not a static representation like a painting or a sculpture, but a moving picture of things, events, processes, ideas, purposes, in which every word is surrounded by a rich penumbra of original concrete experiences, and every sentence brings with it some degree of novelty.

The three worlds of psychological reality evolve gradually with development and experience, ever warped by deficiencies and disturbances in maturation. The overprotected adolescent never learns to use his own senses; the favored one becomes unduly optimistic; the frustrated one takes a gloomy view of life. Each individual tends to color reality in accordance with his own feelings formed during childhood but not overcome by experience. A distorted sense of reality impairs the effectiveness and enjoyment of work and life, creates misunderstanding among people, produces insecurity and inferiority and the resultant frustration. The objective world is a sort of Rorschach inkblot into which each type of adolescent reads a meaning only remotely derived from the shape and color of the blot itself.

The status of the external world transcends all imperfections in the adolescents' perceptions, hence the contrast between the reality of the objective world, on the one hand, and the subjectivity of perceptual experience with their personal bias and distortion, on the other. The world is given but once—not one existing and one perceived, for subject and object are always one. The ego maintains the sense of reality by keeping intact the barrier between the personality and the outside world. It cannot allow the barrier to diminish for a single moment; when the individual loses identity and fuses with the external world, he becomes psychotic. The ego is also the only part of the personality in contact with the outside world, hence it controls perception and feels all actions in the world.

Adolescent derealization is a disturbance of perception of the surrounding real world. The perceptual disorder is accompanied by a feeling of alternation, alienation, unnaturalness, irreality of familiar objects, of living beings and of spatial relationships. Lack of the sense of reality is so marked that everything appears as if through a frosty haze; the trees look as if painted; things seem unreal, dead; somehow all things are the same but not the same. There is a changed perception of time, loss of visual and auditory perception, taste alteration, spatial orientation. The diverse derealization experiences may be accompanied by emotional disorder, depression, dejection. Transient derealization experienced in healthy adolescents is protective to shield the nervous cells from stress.

Lack of Ego Identity

The adolescent gradually develops an accurate, expanding but stable concept about his very self. This self-awareness brings in its train somber companions—fear, anxiety and death awareness. It embodies both a physical and psychological self-image about his capabilities and weaknesses, his expectations from society and what it can expect from him, his notions about the sexual role in the social world for his eventual formulation of a life plan. The transition from dependence to independence is difficult because of the great number of possibilities ahead. It takes trial and error to achieve the tasks of choice via experimentation by word, by deed and in fantasy. Experimentation creates conflict between adolescent and adult with altruistic behavior one morning and greedy behavior the next; perceptive activity one moment and total tolerance the next; frequent shifts in occupational aspirations one time and arguing for asceticism at other times. All this paradoxical behavior is perpetuated with passion and purpose while parents take adolescents at their word, forgetting the duplicity of their intent. Life is a paradox; every truth has its counterpart which contradicts it. As a whole, the adolescent has a serious overall purpose even though day to day processes fluctuate.

We are born unequal and different, yet every adolescent conceals his uniqueness to gain acceptance by peers. He struggles for detachment from parental authority, strives for freedom from the parental bond to establish a sense of identity apart from them, and remains disengaged from society with an inner feeling of noncommitment. He explores his role in society during this psychosocial moratorium, analyzing the faults, inconsistencies and difficulties of the world. He is bewildered by the rapid social changes outmoding his parent as a model for him; by geographic mobility displacing familial cultural models; by classlessness striving to upgrade social status; by blurring of traditional distinction between the sexes. He is bound to ask, "Who am I? What is my role in life to be? Whom do I wish to be like?" A boy's major concerns are self-direction, achievement, authority, sex power; a girl's are appearance, popularity, friendship, dating and sex control. A boy finds his identity through the development of his own competence and his independence in handling work with some promise of achievement; a girl, through the development of close attachments, discovers her own individuality gradually until she has gained security in a stable love relationship.

The power of positive identity is the foundation of personality. It brings the future within adolescent reach as part of his conscious life plan. It establishes the stability of his personality as pictured by himself and his peers; it affirms his stance on who he is. Such self-respect will keep him from being abject when he is in the power of enemies—real or imagined—and will enable him to feel that he may be in the right when the world appears against him. Adolescents unable to measure up conceal their shortcomings from themselves so that the model level of self-esteem is comfortably high. Identity formation is not only a developmental issue but a social issue in our country of heterogeneous races, colors, creeds which can make youth starve as much from lack of self-realization as from lack of bread.

Personal identity is finally achieved with realization of the abstract values that cement human relationships, such as love, honor, loyalty, respect, confidence, charity. This abstract dimension in life enables youth to become his own parent and assume responsibilities for himself with mature understanding. It provides him with a solidarity of being and a stability of purpose. He learns to rely on himself as the primary source of initiative and direction. He fails to abide when adults stand by to oversee his behavior but insists on making, organizing and implementing his own decisions. He pleads for more responsibility and more recognition of his growing self-reliance and prefers to act independently of his parents' desire; nevertheless, he tends to respond because the source of motivation is the parent. He achieves self-determination when self-motivated without depending on others for any impetus. The immature adolescent, however, remains unstable unless he is given individualized therapy to bolster his weaknesses and augment his developmental status to stand on his own feet and act his own unique self. At every moment of life one is what one is going to be, no less than what one has been.

Negative identity or identity diffusion may develop from an inability of the adolescent ego to establish a positive identity. It becomes manifest when youth is barraged with several demands simultaneously, i.e. physical intimacy not necessarily sexual, occupational choice, energetic competition, and/or psychosocial self-definition. He is exposed to age mates from different backgrounds at college or at work while suffering inner conflicts, avoids crucial decisions and is left with outer isolation and inner vacuum. This leads to transitory regression to older involvements in an effort to maintain minimal choice with maximum conviction of being the chooser. He shuns playful intimacy with age mates of both sexes, isolates himself, resorts to stereotyped relations or ventures experiences with odd types. He loses the capacity to abandon himself in sex, turns to a leader to guide him in the art of lovemaking, fails to achieve satisfaction for himself or his confused partner and retreats shamefully in despair. Eventually, there is loss of identity with rejection of ethnic origin, social class, nationality or sexual role. A broken hand works, but not a broken heart.

Lack of Social Activity

Parent desatellization begins at puberty when parents are replaced with glamorous figures for identification. Parents are deemed imperfect but the search for perfect persons is doomed to failure. The task of pseudo-control over adolescent behavior is formidable and may never be achieved, but it must begin at puberty with parental love, tolerance and understanding. Youth's social emergence into an unfamiliar personal world reveals his pattern of personality; the ascetic youth becomes a pillar of virtue in a wicked world; the cynic becomes completely disillusioned and outdoes adult immorality. Whatever the impact, every adolescent questions parental authority and becomes skeptical, argumentative and negativistic. He demands privacy—remains indignant about anyone opening his mail, looking into his wardrobe, and eavesdropping on telephone calls. In his crude striving for total independence, he veers from his confused parents into a world of understanding peers, away from society until ready to accept it with aplomb.

All adolescents belong in different subgroups within their society, each subgroup formed around a nuclear set of values. The peer group offers a sense of belonging essential for maintaining a stable self-concept. Acceptance by the group means acceptance of group values that affect status among peers. With his aspirations for primary status still thwarted, he turns to his peer group for status in the face of intense competitiveness. His reverence is good for nothing if it does not begin with self-respect. The struggle for selfhood is the struggle for independence from adult opinions. Caught in the struggle between independent and dependent strivings, he turns to the peer group for support. This becomes a source of parental anxiety and triggers violent reactions. As he gives up closeness to parents, his aloneness makes him more receptive to the influence of his peers because satisfactory achievement has the highest correlation with personal progress. He conforms assiduously because nonconformists are aggressively sought out for rejection.

Adolescents tend to conform to their own age group in speech, appearance, manners, dress and values because of inferiority and anxiety about personal adequacy. Boys are dominated by the peer group, while girls identify with their own sex before they master the confidence and courage to develop a close relationship with a boy. Crushes involve hero worship, a search for the ideal self and sex idols, a flight after the unattainable. Intense attachments fade once a foundation for a deep relationship with a member of the opposite sex emerges. It is incumbent upon the community to provide opportunities for adolescents to find satisfying safe outlets for their social, emotional and recreational needs, and for parents to provide guidance respectfully, not authoritatively, for authority can rarely survive in face of doubt.

The experienced adolescent gradually acquires rules of conduct necessary and sufficient to insure his ability to live amicably with society as an accepted adult. The social pattern becomes the guide for self-control in adhering to the ethical system of his choice with greater capacity to experience, balance and control emotions by adherence to philosophical principles. Youth gradually develops feelings of tenderness, consideration and respect for others with reciprocity in interpersonal relationships. He gains his own ends without trampling on others' rights to achieve them. He appreciates people as individuals not just objects to use for personal satisfaction. All relationships become more intimate with greater understanding of contemporaries during establishment and fulfillment of appropriate sexual identity.

The social life of the immature youth is one long postponement. He remains a loser and cultivates a solicitude for things rather than people. He rarely gets together with any one of his peers, and then only to do things together in a parallel, not a perpendicular way. But at the heart of his limited social relations, there lurks a hostility momentarily cured but recurring by fits and starts. The great goal is not fulfillment but adjustment; a goal that serves as the maladjustment's weapon. Adapt or perish and/or mingle or fail is nature's inexorable imperative. The immature cannot even fulfill this social obligation to embody the anesthetizing security of poor identification. He regards his own limited life and that of his fellow creatures as meaningless and therefore becomes disqualified for life unless adequate maturation is fully provided under medical supervision.

Lack of Individual Freedom

Man is not born free. At the moment of birth he is the helpless prey of his reflexes and the passive recipient of conditions imposed on him by his family and his culture. He can exercise no initiative and make no decisions. His education is a slow induction into the possibilities of freedom with a transfer of restraint from the outer world to the inner self. It gives him a progressive increase of choice as intelligence, experience and imagination widen the range of his vision and increase the possible alternatives before him. Increasing selectivity and increasing self-direction are the rewards of youth's capacity for freedom. It cannot be granted; it is something the adolescent takes according to maturity. It is inconsequential to know how to free himself, the arduous thing is to know what to do with his freedom since there is no apprenticeship for freedom. It is the faculty that enlarges the usefulness of all other faculties. Everything great is created by the individual who can labor in freedom, yet it is not good to be too free; it is not good to have everything one wants.

Every ubiquitous adolescent is devoted to issues of emancipation, independence and freedom from the family, the crucial pre-

lude to becoming a separate being. There may be open rebellion,
rejection of home standards, resentment against parents, or withdrawal, secrecy and privacy, especially among girls. Adolescents
want but fear independence for they still have deep emotional
ties to their family and yearn for the love and protection of early
childhood. This ambivalence about independence further produces provocative behavior as a bid for parental attention, but
youth may assume outer defenses of bravado, boredom or playing
it cool, and remain very sensitive to criticism. Adolescents are
sure to be losers when they battle with themselves; it is a civil
war where triumphs are defeats.

The adolescent always fears to go to the end of his thoughts.
He is not free; he does not feel free. Freedom is an irksome burden unless the youth has talents to make something of himself.
Emancipation from the bondage of the soil is not freedom for
the tree. The misfortune which befalls the adolescent from his
once having been a child is that his liberty was at first concealed
from him, and all his life he retains the nostalgia for the time
when he was ignorant of the exigencies. The free way of life
proposes ends but it does not prescribe means. Every phase of
life rests on the reconciliation of the opposite states: necessity
and freedom, stabilization and change, security and adventure.
Without regularity there would not be enough constancy in life
to enable one to recognize change itself for good or bad.

Hierarchic organization in the adolescent and in society creates
conditions favorable to freedom: release from automatism to give
him a greater degree of self-direction after a long childhood of
bondage to parents. But freedom does not mean the casting-off
of restraints, destruction, inhibition, or the denial of duties and
responsibilities. An adolescent loses his freedom through poverty,
ignorance, immaturity, disease, overdevelopment of a single organ function or overcommitment to social processes. But he
fights to establish independence from adults by rebelling against
adult domination, by resenting interference with his plans, by
veering away from home more and more, by engaging in secret
activities, by choosing his own friends, by behavior according to
shifting peer codes, by identifying with his own sex. Youth feels

so rich in his opportunities for free expression that he often no longer knows what he is free from; nor does he know where he is not, and does not recognize his native autocrats when he sees them.

The age of the adolescent is a direct function of the degree of freedom accorded. If these privileges have occurred with growth, there is positive evidence of progress. That's the lot of the normal child teeming with progress. "Unto every one that hath shall be given—but from him that hath not shall be taken away." In the course of development, no child has ever been made a present of freedom. It has a high price; and every youngster must show his mettle and struggle to preserve it. The very idea of freedom rests on a profound respect for humanity. It is deeply religious, ethical and moral in its basis. It is better for youth to deserve freedom without receiving than to receive without deserving. After all, youth tends towards a straight path and strives innately by that which is born in him. Yet the feeling that life is meaningless, that the world is not going anywhere in particular, that man is an insignificant part in the scheme of things haunts every youth. Some take refuge in traditional religions, others escape into blatant hedonism, still others take the easiest way and settle on raising a family. That was meaningful to the primitive, to the common youth, but not to the uncommon youth. In reality, human natures form a spectrum ranging from the most common to the most uncommon. And every community is renewed out of the unknown common ranks and not out of established uncommon individuals.

Lack of Heterosexual Interest

The feeling of apartness from others comes to most with puberty, but it is not always developed to such a degree as to make the difference between the individual and his fellows so noticeable to the normal individual. But the immature adolescent remains apart in timidity, for immature is the love of youth and immature his hatred of man. The wings of his youthful spirit are still tied down. He is strong in body, weak in mind, nondescript in sex, but very certain about everything and yet able to use nothing. He possesses sexual organs but her sexual organs possess woman. The sex identification by parents will determine his sexual behavior, i.e. the identification masculine or feminine, the psychological gender the same as the biological. Our society is growing more feminine as it grows more complex. The adolescent must develop his biologic sex to the fullest with members of the opposite sex to neutralize any subnormal sex identification. The capacity to relate to other beings with constancy involves sustained friendship, a direct function of absent ambivalence, i.e. mixed feelings, love, hate, fear, acquired from early object relations. But the greater the boy's attachment to his mother, the more difficult, for in such separation he loses part of himself. Amoebas at the start were not complex; they tore themselves apart and started sex. Man's sexuality pervades his whole life, commencing in late adolescence to find one outer place in the wider world, and another inner place for intimacy with the opposite sex.

The sexual drive in the adolescent male is simple; its propagative function under androgen control and discharge involves a single act and the urgency of his sexual impulses is a direct function of gonadal hormone production. But in the female, there is a cycle of recessions and reintegrations of the psychosexual pattern. The sexual cycle begins with the ripening of the follicle, and the estrogen secreted mobilizes active heterosexual manifestations, expressed by conscious or disguised desires and by increased alertness in extroverted activities. The heterosexual need parallels the increasing estrogen production, reaching its height at the time of ovulation and the heightened sexuality during adolescence is strongly influenced by psychological changes. In boys, the sex drive tends to be biological, direct and impersonal. In girls, sexuality is repressed to be expressed in romantic dreams of love. The earlier masturbation of girls adds to the difficulties between the sexes as does the greater social skill of girls.

The substance of young men's lives is woman. All other things are irrelevancies, hypocrisies, subterfuges. They sit talking of sports, politics, careers, and all the while their hearts are filled with thoughts of women and the conquest of women. What would youth be without love? Love enters man through his eyes and nose, i.e. through sight and smell; and woman through the ears and mind, i.e. voice and memory. Man has his will but woman has her way. But it is the man who gives charm to womanhood, that provides a glow to her face, softness in her voice, and a grace in her motions. The sexual horizon of youth is determined by ego, rearing and associations. The older boy or girl usually has some heterosexual association, judging from the attraction to specific individuals of the opposite sex. The adolescent girl behaves more understandingly about sex, begins to use cosmetics, knows whom she likes at school and criticizes most of the boys for their behavior. Actual interest in a peer of the opposite sex is far more significant than any presumed sexual intercourse. A boy's reserved statement that he has never had a real date with a girl may really mean that he does not have the automobile facilities to carry on sexually.

The older adolescent gradually accepts himself as a sexually mature person for meaningful heterosexual relationships. Physical changes during puberty are so rapid that he is not fully able to integrate or adjust to them. And so he questions everything as he beholds his bodily changes, critical of his complexion, height, weight, body pattern, facial features, teeth or anything about him or within him. There is a compelling preoccupation with physical appearance; the girl in front of the mirror, and the boy in the gymnasium workout. Once secondary sex characteristics appear there is a personal yearning for physical sameness with contemporaries for developmental acceleration or retardation causes anxiety; and delayed sexual development causes anguish. Both boys and girls with belated physical maturation are exposed to different socio-psychological environments with adverse effects. Sex drives become more urgent with the concomitant increase in the need for sexual outlet via masturbation, evanescent sexual experiences with others of the same sex, heterosexual activity and actual sexual intercourse. Satisfactory heterosexual relationships are achieved by increased contact, more dating, extensive discussion, sexual fantasy, physical exploration and personal experimentation. The ultimate objective is to solidify the personal sexual role and yet enjoy sexual feelings.

The immature youth lacks heterosexual interest and avoids intimacies not to expose his inadequacy. He is full of misinformation on sexual matters and builds up a barrage of self-defense against involvement with a member of the opposite sex. But once the underlying endocrine basis of emotional deviation is brought to relatively normal levels, the whole spectre of sex interest and relationship changes. At best, many years are wasted in social preliminaries before any positive biological reaction is effected with a member of the other sex. Experience between the sexes is in the fingers and head; the heart remains inexperienced. What is intersexual experience? A poor little hut built from the ruins of the golden palace called illusions. The advantaged youth has a difficult but luxurious choice of opportunities; but the disadvantaged and immature youth has only two choices—to accept social rejection and educational and occupational failure in a pattern of fatalism and passivity, or to lash out violently against the society which condemns him to inferiority, deprivation and humiliation.

Lack of Vocational Vision

Youth is the time to do something and be somebody. The bitter and the sweet come from the outside; the hard from within, from one's own efforts. Despite the success cult, adolescents are most deeply moved not by reaching a goal, but by exerting the effort involved in getting there—or failing to get there. But effort is only effort when it begins to hurt; by labor, fire is gotten out of a stone. The test of a vocation is the love of drudgery it involves. Youth is never well but in action, and then he feels immortal. Every kind of work—intellectual or manual—is sacred and gives peace of mind. When youth is rightly occupied, ambivalence grows out of the work, as the color petals out of a fruitful flower. Work is the meat of life, pleasure the dessert.

Youth must love and work, for all work is empty save when there is love. If the work of youth is to succeed, it must spring from within him, not be imposed upon him from without. There are three tests of wise choice of suitable work: it must be honest, useful, and cheerful. The time will come when every kind of work will be judged by two measurements: one by the product itself, as is now done, and the other by the effect of the work on the producer. To give satisfaction, work should not be too mechanical or too monotonous. The work should make one feel that his productivity is worthwhile; it should allow some play for individuality, taste and creativity; it should offer companionship among peers at work; it should be correlated with scientific knowledge to advance the outlook in the field. The happy adolescent is he who likes his work, for all education is a fraud if it turns out people who don't like their work.

The choice of a vocation must not be left to chance. "What sort of job am I fitted for? What are my natural abilities?" The adolescent must ask these questions. Natural abilities are like natural plants that need pruning by study. In a world as empirical as ours, an adolescent who does not know what he is good at will not be sure what he is good for. Blessed is he who has found his work. What a travesty on time that the only thing a man can do for eight hours a day, day after day, is work. You can't eat eight hours, nor drink for eight hours a day, nor make love for eight hours, nor play for eight hours. Yet the master-word for youth looms large in meaning. It is the open sesame to every portal, the great equalizer in the world, the true philosopher's stone which transmutes all the base metal of humanity into gold. And, the master-word is work at a vocation of choice.

The immature adolescent remains totally dependent upon parents without seeking any preparation for a livelihood. It is a personality weakness that leads to lifelong degradation. Youth seeks answers to questions within himself, finds nothing beyond his short range of experience and concludes that there is nothing outside himself, either. He is not the youngster to seek an after-school job to help support the family and enhance his maturation economically, socially and emotionally. Experience in earning money for services rendered is invaluable in the practical outlook towards a vocation. An adolescent may change his mind about the kinds of life endeavor to follow but the very thinking about a life work is a forward step. The immature adolescent not only lacks ability to cultivate a life vocation but does not have the inner drive to achieve any objective. He goes along under home prodding, barely gets by at school or at play, and remains unnoticed on the sidelines. It is imperative to evaluate his potential abilities in order to transform them into a suitable vocation to earn his own livelihood in order to protect his freedom, his independence and self-respect. It will enable him to feel that he may be in the right when the world is against him; how else can he be comfortable without his own approval? He can be made comfortable by easing the stress and overcoming the immaturity.

Emotional stress and/or immaturity impinging on the adolescent releases three clusters of dysfunction: physical or psychosomatic affecting one or more organs; mood changes; behavior disorders. Disturbed adolescents thus reveal functional and organic disorders, hence the need for medical evaluation before psychiatric intervention. This is particularly true of patients with multiple psychosomatic complaints, because of the lengthening of the adolescent period, affluence, urbanization, rapid shifts in moral standards, and the rising complexity of vocational opportunities. Even the best young people are stumbling on the threshold of adulthood burdened by problems they cannot solve alone. Many of the desperate adolescents turn to medical and psychotherapeutic help. Some seek treatment on their own, others come reluctantly. But youth can be frustrating, ever-persisting in their maladaptive behavior. Evincing personal interest in youth and his problems enables treatment of the patient and his disorders. Transference gives the patient confidence in the physician and counter-transference returns this feeling of affection toward the patient to displace the cool feeling about doctors. Ventilation relieves the patient of emotional tension. Medication corrects emotional disturbance when the physician has complete control of the situation involving adolescent, parents, peers and teachers.

Disturbed immature adolescents are remarkably vulnerable and remarkably treatable. They are flexible, impressionable, elastic and resilient but also brittle when hit too hard. They often break into bizarre behavior yet are malleable enough to return to conventional appearance with gentle patient handling. Immature youth is usually in a mood to talk, to discuss values, motivations, ethics, life, death, suicide. They are eager for guidance when directed by those who can bring order out of chaos without super-imposing conformity with family patterns. Such youth wants help for self-expression in the light of his own limited objectives rather than to be molded by those who have preconceived ideas of how young people should behave. If short-term therapy is offered in this spirit, the immature adolescent responds in a gratifying manner. He accepts interpretations with interest and curiosity without being frightened by them. His behavior and his degree of happiness often change markedly for the better after short periods of vocational guidance.

Lack of Emotional Communication

How to manage the adolescent? Home administration, like a machine, does not create. It just carries on. But parents must oil the works for smooth operations day after day, without breakdown in interrelations. Bad administration can destroy good policy but good administration can never save bad policy. As in all areas of human adjustment there are no absolute rules, only good principles to apply with respect. Precision of communication is most important in this era of hair-trigger balances, when a misunderstood word or feeling may create as much disaster as a sudden thoughtless act. Parents seek pitifully to convey to adolescents the treasures of their hearts, but youths have not the power to accept them. And so both go lonely, side by side, but not together; parents unable to know youth and unknown by them. After all, youth finds room in a few square inches of his face for the traits of all his ancestors, for the expression of all his history, and his current needs and wants. When his eyes say one thing and his tongue another, an understanding parent relies on the language of the eyes for face-saving fruitful sessions.

Parents must resort to sanity, soundness and sincerity in communicating with youth. Both will flourish in a culture of clarification. The elders should retreat in the background with obscurity and competence to give youth some of the limelight for experience that comes in good stead in the world without. More time should be spent with adolescents, more things should be done with them, more leeway should be given them—all with a good sense of humor, none with argumentation. Compromise may not be the spice of life but it is its solidity. It is always better to lose the saddle than the horse. In compromise there is an adjustment of conflicting interests to give each adversary the satisfaction of thinking he has got what he ought not to have, and is deprived of nothing except what was justly his due. Blessed are the peacemakers to free themselves from painful wrath.

Parental kindness has never weakened the stamina or softened the fiber of youth. Parents don't have to be cruel to be tough. Nothing is so strong as gentleness, and nothing is so gentle as real strength. A sweet tongue, courtesy and gentleness will guide an elephant with a hair. The great parent knows the power of gentleness and only uses force when persuasion fails. An adolescent needs much praise but it should be reasonable and honest. Praise is the best diet for us. After all, youth needs much reassurance from parents about his basic capacities, talents, attractiveness. Such praise solidifies the parent-adolescent bond, gives the adolescent self-esteem. Such self-respect enhanced by wise parental understanding of youth will keep him from being abject when he is in the power of enemies—real or virtual—and will enable him to feel that he may be in the right when the world is against him. All criticism should be tactful, constructive and firm and always coupled with an honest compliment to soften resentment. Adolescents are ready to suffer anything from parents or from Heaven itself, provided that when it comes to words, they are untouched.

Liberty for youth means responsibility. That is why it is dreaded. Too little liberty brings stagnation; too much brings chaos. The adolescent is forever seeking more liberty; sometimes the request is reasonable, more often it is out of bounds. The best approach is to couple liberty with responsibility. It buffers the rate of assumption of liberty when it is too fast. An adolescent is either free or he is not; there is no apprenticeship for freedom. Unless he has talents to make something of himself, freedom is an irksome burden. He prates of freedom when he is in deadly fear of life. To know how to free himself is nothing; the arduous thing is to know what to do with his freedom. To become a man is precisely to be responsible. Indeed, there is no growth except in the fulfillment of all obligations. Parental good intentions are useless in the absence of common sense. Nothing astonishes youth so much as common sense and plain dealing. It is the shortest time between two points that applies good judgment, sound discretion and practical wisdom.

EMOTIONAL MATURATION

Youth is composed of immature individuals dominated by disordered infantile patterns of feeling, thinking and behavior. Primary developmental forces reestablish the earlier patterns; secondary emotional forces condition the personality by training, imitation, identification and experience; tertiary emotional forces adapt the being for survival amidst the realities of the world and the exactions of body and mind. These three forces lead to maturity circuitously to achieve optimal functioning and full enjoyment of adult powers. Maturation consists of the gradual development of innate capacities, independent of learning, training or experience. The process of maturation ripens these innate potentialities into capacities for specific behavior. This growth from within produces peculiarities of temperament which determine youth's ability to acquire new forms of behavior for everyday adjustment.

Emotional maturation promotes greater feeling, motivating and reacting to one's self and to other beings. Emotions are endless; the more youth expresses them, the more he may have to express. And so the course of emotional maturation proceeds of its own accord with the environment supplying the essential stimulating conditions. It is very much like a pine tree that grows strong and tall, if provided with proper soil, climate, protection and freedom. The proper conditions provided by nature equate with loving understanding of human needs. If conditions are favorable, youth develops positive feelings for and identification with persons closest to him. But parental feelings create cumulative tensions from the time a soft baby is precipitated into a hard world. These early emotional reactions determine the attitudes, modes and fixations of life, and the resulting personality distortions emerge from the methods adopted by the child to cope with the needs, conflicts and problems that arouse intolerable anxiety at home.

The emotional mind is molded during the first six years. A child's feelings towards parents and siblings so formed persist throughout life as the permanent nucleus in the evolution of personality. The childishness in us lives on even though the personality matures. A child treated negatively during this period reacts with constant hostility against others and himself. The negative feelings may be overlaid by friendliness later in childhood, but the pattern of maturing has been warped just as the sapling that is crushed and bent yet matures growing towards the sun. It is never quite as strong a tree for having been bent as a twig. The person with loving feelings towards parents and siblings, disturbed by fright, fear and hostility during the first six years of life, will never be emotionally healthy as an adult. The pattern of disturbed emotional relations developed during the early formative years is the key to psychopathology with a whole range of emotional disorders from invisible inner suffering to criminal behavior. Adolescent behavior becomes intelligible only in terms of his reactions as a child determined by the way he was treated. Wolves and hawks could teach humans about proper parenthood and peaceful relations with one's own kind. The final test of emotional maturity is to live with fear and not be afraid, to laugh at one's self when the need to defend one's self is minimal; to acquire the ideal self one would like to be, even though the actual self does not measure up to this ideal.

Emotional Maturation Tests and Measurements

Alexander, T.: The prediction of teacher-pupil interaction with a projective test. *J. Clin. Psychol.*, 6:273, 1950.
Aronfreed, J. et al.: *The Concept of Internalization, Handbook of Internalization Theory.* New York, Rand McNally, 1967.
Aronfreed, J.: *Conduct and Conscience: The Socialization of Internalized Control Over Behavior.* New York, Academic Press, 1968.
Bandura, A. et al.: *Adolescent Aggression.* New York, Ronald Press, 1959.

Bell, G. D.: Process in the formation of adolescents' aspirations. *Social Forces, 42:*178, 1963.

Cervantes, L. F.: *The Dropout.* Ann Arbor, University of Michigan Press, 1965.

Cohen, A. K.: The sociology of the deviant act: anomie theory and beyond. *Am. Sociol. Rev., 30:*5, 1965.

Cromwell, R. L. *et al.:* Behavior classification of emotionally disturbed children. Paper read at Council of Exceptional Children, Portland, Oregon, 1965.

Douvan, E. *et al:* Modal patterns in American adolescence. *Review of Child Development Research.* New York, Russell Sage Foundation, 1966.

Engle, M.: The stability of the self concept in adolescence. *J. Abnorm. Soc. Psychol., 58:*211, 1959.

Fuller, E. M.: How do children feel about it? *Childhood Educ., 23:*124, 1956.

Goffman, E.: *The Presentation of Self in Everyday Life.* New York, Double-day-Anchor, 1959.

Grusec, J.: Some antecedents of self-criticism. *J. Pers. Soc. Psychol., 4:*244, 1966.

Hirschfield, P. P.: Response set in impulsive children. *J. Genet. Psychol., 107:*117, 1965.

Horrocks, J. E.: *The Psychology of Adolescence.* New York, Houghton Mifflin, 1962.

Kohlberg, L. *et al.:* Development of moral character and moral ideology. *Child Development Research.* New York, Russell Sage Foundation, 1964, Vol. I.

Koppitz, E. M.: Emotional indicators on human figure drawings in children. A validation study. *J. Clin. Psychol., 22:*313, 1966.

Lore, R. K.: Palmar sweating and transitory anxiety in children. *Child Dev., 37:* 115, 1966.

Maas, H. S.: The role of members in clubs of lower-class and middle-class adolescents. *Child Dev., 25:*241, 1954.

McClosky, H. *et al.:* Psychological dimensions of anomie. *Am. Soc. Rev., 30:* 14, 1965.

Piers, E. V. *et al.:* Age and other correlates of self-concept in children. *J. Educ. Psychol., 55:*91, 1964.

Rubin, E. Z. *et al.: Emotionally Handicapped Children and the Elementary School.* Detroit, Wayne State University Press, 1966.

Strauss, A. A. *et al.:* Behavior differences in mentally retarded children measured by a new behavior rating scale. *Am. J. Psychiatry, 96:*1117, 1940.

Verville, E.: *Behavior Problems of Children.* Philadelphia, Saunders, 1967.

Winker, J. B.: Age trends and sex differences in the wishes, identification, activities, and fears of children. *Child Dev., 20:*91, 1949.

Wylie, R.: *The Self-Concept.* Lincoln, University of Nebraska Press, 1961.

Emotional Processes

Emotion moves youth to love, to fight, to run away—but it also moves them to think. The immature individual remains a dullard, much readier to feel and digest than to think and consider. No emotion any more than a wave can long retain its individual form in him. Feeling and emotion are natural responses to stimuli which dramatize the dynamics of behavior, enrich life and give meaning to existence. Life should be very drab without love, pleasure, excitement, wonder and other such positive feelings. Even the more disruptive feelings like anger, fear and anxiety energize responses for security, safety and accomplishment. Feelings like admiration, respect, reverence, sorrow and remorse transform the pale facade of existence into vibrant living. Without pride and passion, sympathy and sorrow, the dull moments of time would tick off as endless eternity of meaningless existence. Once an emotion is launched it never disappears from the body; strong ones linger for months. The secret of life is never to have an emotion that is unbecoming.

The brain has 10 billion nerve cells for the intellectual mind and 2 billion for the emotional mind, transmitting messages to each other by low-watt electricity. Intellect works with an inner calm but emotion with an inner turmoil. Both harbor lifelong reactions in every speck of the brain via the ceaseless dance of molecules. Emotion really means inner turbulence. It cannot be delineated into love, hate, fear, anger, for each distinction is a mirage existing only in the eye of the beholder. Separating one emotion from another is like packaging mists. Arrogance masks insecurity, humility disguises arrogance. Emotions are only sand dunes, so shiftable that they are unworthy of special names. The problem is to understand the desert and the prevailing winds and act accordingly. Psychologists acknowledge four emotions; patients describe 500; but Jung divided beings into extroverts and introverts, although everyone is a combination of both.

Emotion can easily get out of hand and precipitate an explosion. It disorganizes thinking and disrupts behavior once anger foils into rage and fear leaps into panic. An isolated incident does not disturb the personality, if limited, but a prolonged period of frustration leads to emotional chaos. Enforced conformity creates angry and defiant feelings, the suppressed feelings are driven internally only to prevent them from ever emerging; while repressed tensions are buried alive, and the neurotic symptoms emanate in disguised form in exchange. If youth is in trouble, come to his aid. Ask yourself: "What is wrong in his life?" If we can stop thinking of an adolescent as good or bad but as learning; if we can interpret our values in terms of understandable thoughts and feelings, the discipline problem will become a constructive process of learning how to live. Discipline is essential for optimal inner peace for optimal emotional development for optimal mental health.

Our culture demands restraint and renunciation, sacrifice and strategy as everyday techniques of self-discipline, yet the spirit of parent-child relationships is more important than the method of discipline. The art vested in the feeling tone behind the relationship is far more significant than the science of disciplinary procedure. It is the kind of feeling that parents transmit to youth rather than the things they do that creates emotional harmony. Democratic home discipline is self-discipline by all members of an harmonious family. It can be very severe; it can be the very opposite of anarchy, but it cannot exist without a feeling of freedom to discuss in the family. The unsuspecting youth is the first to profit by such democratic decorum.

Self-understanding is essential for adolescent understanding. Parents must have acceptance of themselves before they can help youth with emotional problems; they must be at peace with themselves before they can influence youth in a wholesome way. St. Francis De Sales pointed this out ages ago, "How can we reprove children gently if we correct ourselves with disgust?" He who frets about his own imperfections cannot correct youth; effective correction can only come from a peaceful mind. Youth evolves a reaction pattern for adaptation: submission, withdrawal or rebellion to maintain a precarious balance between the struggle to maintain his individuality in the face of disturbing attitudes and the struggle to preserve his place in his parents' affection.

Youth compromises himself to maintain security in the face of abnormal attitudes even if it warps his emotions.

Emotional disturbance arises from an abnormal attitude or action towards youth by some member of the family significant in his life. The primary abnormality is not in the adolescent but in the emotionally charged interaction between him and a parent. Outer manifestations reflect a disturbed bond or a difficult personality makeup that stirs a negative response in the sensitive parent. The abnormal behavior can be corrected at its inception if the cause is recognized but it cannot be altered by threats, sedation or manipulation. It is well to unravel youth's relationships with those around him. Once the cause of the behavior is understood and modified, the emotional difficulty diminishes or disappears. Parental rejection, obvious or disguised, may be a disturbing force in the life of the adolescent. The attitude threatens his feeling of security and sense of worth, i.e. excessive parental demands beyond innate capacities precipitate neurotic reactions; rigid enforcement of unrealistic regulations creates emotional discord. Parental overprotection is as detrimental as underprotection in emotional health, i.e. the parent who fights youth's battle is depriving him of the privilege of maturation by experience and the parent who has no control over youth is cultivating an egocentric, emotionally unstable tyrant. Some parents blow hot and cold, overprotective one time and underprotective another, only to create emotional confusion.

Emotional Control

There is a raging tiger inside every adolescent but every man worthy of the respect of his children spends his life building inside for himself a cage to pen that tiger in. And every youth becomes a king when he learns how to rule himself. Emotional health can be cultivated by learning to control feelings. Enthronement of feeling leads to dethronement of reason, for reason is the only source of control of internal responses. When feeling achieves overwhelming power, freedom declines. Reasoning is a powerful technique but the language of reason is too cold and too slow to make the necessary impression. It will have no effect on the understanding, because it does not stir adolescent feeling unless reason is inculcated at every turn. Without real understanding desirable action is impossible. Even the language of kindness unassociated with reason will be unable to persuade, because it lacks conviction. But reason and kindness united in discourse will rarely be resisted by an affable youth in a calm atmosphere. The tendency to exalt intuition and to deprecate intellect is an unworthy retreat from reason. Youth needs both for effective discipline. The well-disciplined youth is the one who is able to intercept at will the communication between the senses and the mind. Emotional symptoms are psychological devices to cope hastily with the demands of reality. And symptom formation is one step removed from neurotic and psychotic development which disintegrate the personality. The adolescent can be taught to solve his problems while maintaining his vital balance, for explosive emotional symptoms serve the subjective demands of feeling rather than objective evidence of reason. We must untangle youth from the skein of his emotions to achieve and maintain an integrated maturation of the total personality.

Youth is potentially a rational being with feelings complemental to his rational nature; reason should, therefore, exercise control over feelings and emotions. Youth must learn to live by reason to lay the groundwork for lifelong mental health. A special kind of mental discipline controls youth's emotions. It is not the kind applied thoughtlessly as a distorted caricature of the real thing—harsh punishment, withheld love, or sadistic criticism creating the fear and anxiety that permeate the life of an army where one fears the other above him, but the harmony that pervades the atmosphere of an orchestra where all work in loving unison. Youth realizes the dangerous implications of loss of emotional control for their own impulses frighten them. Conflicts with parents and authorities disturb them into the realization that the only antidote is disciplinary existence. Emotional anarchy arises from sexual impulses when feelings get out of hand and guilt becomes unbearable with anxiety and confusion about present events and future possibilities. Some adolescents have disturbed homosexual tendencies that erupt into destructive personality relationships; some reveal unbridled hostility difficult to control, with rebellion against parents, resistance to society and revolt against religion. It precipitates depression, despair or self-destruction, reversed only by self-discipline.

Wholesome values guide human reason in coping with the demands and hardships, the tragedies and frustrations of daily life. To know what is good and worthwhile and to strive actively for it is as important to healthy emotions as good food, fresh air and exercise are to the physique. Youth can and must be taught to develop healthy attitudes towards self, towards others, towards reality, towards life, towards God. There is no room in the healthy mind for cynicism, pessimism and other isms that poison thoughts without positive replacements. Youth needs optimal development of spiritual resources: courage, patience, compassion, fortitude, charity and temperance. There are times when it becomes necessary to reestablish the primacy of reason because feeling has gained the upper hand and control has largely disappeared. Every youth can be taught emotional control by deliberate acts of will and wisdom via training, education and treatment. Emotional deviations can be reversed from wretched childhood into resourceful maturity. The capacity and desire to develop potentialities are inherent in every being for man can change and go on changing as long as he lives.

Conscience stores the do's and don'ts from parental indoctrination. It is the internal Hall of Justice that holds youth accountable for the things he does. It is the mother, father, police and judge who molds the ideals of his "self." It is mind's battlefield where the internal civil war is fought to preserve personal union with or against his family. It is here that youth struggles with feelings, right and wrong, true and false, good and evil, shame and guilt, tyranny and oppression. It is here that his rebellion begins to triumph, to flounder, or to end in shame, humiliation and self-punishment. The emotionally stable youth reveals attitudes discernible in the way he regards himself and others. He has a good opinion of himself. He neither denies nor overestimates himself but always sees room for self-improvement. His sense of humor makes him view himself objectively and permits him to be amused at his own foibles. He sees the absurdity that often exists in human situations but does not condemn others for the weaknesses that create such situations. Such an emotionally stable adolescent enjoys the company of others and respects them whether he likes them or not. He refuses to permit emotional prejudices to come between him and his fellow-man and never sits in judgment of them. He sometimes disapproves of what they do but feels no unhealthy compulsion to tell them so unless it is his duty to do so. He does not actively dislike people for their faults, knowing full well that one can hate the sin and love the sinner.

The emotionally mature adolescent enjoys work, play and cooperative activity with others. He learns not to be lonely by himself for he can use privacy for reflection. Other people's opinions are important to him but they do not alarm him if not approved. Nevertheless, he weighs criticism objectively, determines its validity and applies it for self-improvement. He does not dwell on criticism nor on the people who make it. The emotionally mature adolescent develops a philosophy of life that helps him to do his best at all times with the help of spiritual values and positive attitudes towards himself, others and society. Such philosophical decisions are the crystallized reflections of common life, methodized and corrected with discretion. A personal philosophy guides him in viewing the world about him, in evaluating current events, in planning his own future, and in making the best possible contribution to his community and country.

Emotional Growth

Youth is a composite of several ages—physical, mental, emotional and social. The closer they are to the chronological age, the more balanced the development, the more stable the personality, the more desirable the behavior. It is essential to recognize the level of each developmental tempo to achieve the proper balance for each age. Once the nature of the deviation is established, every effort must be made to correct it for optimal body balance for optimal personality functioning. Everything that grows follows a ground-plan laid down at its inception.

Out of this planned matrix arises each phase of the being with its own timetable for optimal development. If a part fails to achieve its maturation at a proper time, the functional harmony of the whole child is affected. In the development of personality there is progressive emergence of emotional control, social capacity, sense of values, and ways of coping with everyday experiences to plunge into the secret of life more deeply than the grownups venture. The dazzling process of inner branching perceived by Erikson involves eight stages of psychic struggles: basic trust vs. mistrust in the infant; autonomy vs. doubt in the toddler; initiative vs. guilt in the preschooler; industry vs. inferiority in the school child; identity vs. confusion in the puberal child; intimacy vs. isolation in the adolescent; generativity vs. stagnation in the young adult; ego integrity vs. despair in the mature being. Each step depends upon fulfillment of the previous step. If one step in the development is accomplished, the next step will proceed satisfactorily; otherwise, the process is arrested, delayed or defective. Man is a born child, his power is the power of growth. There are few successful adolescents who were not first successful children nurtured by wholesome parents.

The adolescent organism reaches the end of its growth but his psychological state remains immature. In our culture, biological growth is ahead of psychological maturation, accounting for most of the peculiarities of the adolescent. The biological ability to procreate is foisted upon an emotionally unprepared organism. A full-grown body is entrusted to an inexperienced mind. The adolescent is awkward and insecure and knows not what to do with himself. He feels as if he were constantly in a test situation to prove to himself and others that he is already a man. The only way to do this is to measure himself against others. The competition demands continuous practice of full-grown capacities to grow emotionally into the mature status already attained biologically several years before. Once youth can take his capacities for granted, his interest no longer centers around the self but around the environment.

The psychological attributes of maturity arise from the balance between intake and retention of substance and energy vs. expenditure. The wish to receive no longer outweighs the wish to give at maturity. Growth ceases; the body can no longer organize more living matter within its own system. The surplus energy is now released for propagation and productive work. The extra energy of the mature person shows itself in generosity—a giver more than a getter. This altruism, the basis of morality, has a biological foundation; but the platonic ideal of emotional maturity is never attained completely; it is only approached. Individual differences are enormous, accounting for the few leaders and many followers. Whenever life becomes difficult for youth there is a tendency to regress to less mature attitudes and rely on parents. In our hearts, we all regret having been expelled from the Garden of Eden having eaten from the tree of knowledge—a symbol of maturity. In crucial life situations, individuals become insecure and seek help long before exhausting all their resources.

Emotional Attachments

Emotional maturation is not a matter of fate or fortune but of parental responsibility. It is possible only if children can form attachments to people of significance to them. The first such relationship is with the mother; the next, with the father or father-substitute; and the next, with siblings and other children. Man is a knot, a web, a mesh into which these relationships are tied, for only these alone matter. Like higher primates, human beings in social groups are under a protective existence for the immature members to mature and learn adult skills. The only significant social group, necessary and sufficient, is the nuclear family unit of father, mother and siblings, even though anthropologically, ethnologically and historically, the nuclear family unit group is not a satisfactory child-rearing unit. In adolescence, the behavior of humans and primates is very similar; pre-puberal boys and girls form peer group attachments and make significant relationships with one of the mothers of the group. Similarly, preadolescent chimpanzees form a group with juvenile and adolescents who move about with one or two mature females. Adolescent

boys need significant attachments to extra-parental male adults
as adolescent chimpanzees need association with mature males.
Psychological maturation in adolescence thus requires a balance
between the individual, the nuclear family, the extra-parental
adults and the peer group. The most significant relationships
essential for the development of identity are attachment: first,
to a parental adult; second, to the peer group; third, to the nuclear family. In preadolescent childhood, the hierarchy attachment is to the nuclear family, peer group and extra-parental adult.
All are necessary, and if one is absent, maturity is impeded. If
man is to survive without polluting his environment and destroy-
ing himself, the population will be limited to a small family
unit with one or two children in emotional isolation. Society
will thus need to recreate tribal society as psychological disintegration increases.

In the Middle Ages, the family was not the only significant
unit for emotional growth. The aristocracy sent adolescents to
other noble houses to be educated while the middle classes
farmed their children out to be skilled as apprentices at puberty.
As attachment to parents grows weaker while other adults and
peers assume primary roles in their lives, psychological maturation during adolescence requires a dynamic balance of meaningful emotional relationships between the individual and his parents, the peer group and the extra-parental adults. The weaker
the social structure, the more significant the attachment to individuals. Such identification with individuals of choice represents a personal development of the concept, "This is who and
what I am." It is present only in the adolescent with the capacity
for making emotional ties with others. Parent, extra-parent and
peer group can become of such emotional significance that absence or premature separation from one or the other may give
rise to the same classical triad associated with premature separation of an infant from its mother, i.e. protest, despair and detachment. If parents are not available to the adolescent he can, nevertheless, develop a sense of autonomy if he still has relationships
with a peer group and with extra-parental adults. A young
adolescent seeks an additional parent substitute tenuously be-

cause the imprint of his parents' relationship remains internalized at puberty.

An adolescent must try to weaken the persistent bond with parents because continuous identification with them binds his perception of their personality with his own and blocks the sense of autonomy. The adolescent who lacks contact with extra-parental adults while weakening the bond with parents needs strong attachments to his peer group. He must have relationships outside the nuclear family to develop a sense of personal autonomy. The generation gap is an inevitable result of the failure of society to provide the opportunity of forming attachment bonds with extra-parental adults. Without such personalized adults, dependence on the unstable peer group, not on stable parents, becomes more intensified. Adolescents over-attached to peers become vulnerable to group contagion by projecting their hostility on the outside world. If neither peer groups nor extra-parental adults are available for attachment bonds, then despair and detachment follow and individual autonomy is doomed to failure. Even healthy adolescents need consistent success with peer groups before they can make significant emotional attachments. The junior high school system makes it difficult for young adolescents to cultivate peer group or extra-parental adult relationships because they are exposed to many daily classes and many different teachers, with five minutes to move from room to room and no recess period for socialization. Our current school situation breeds emotional detachment with consequent withdrawal to the nuclear family.

Psychologically disturbed adolescents who are unable to establish relationships with anyone but their parents require psychotherapy. They cannot mature in isolation, hence children in Russia and Israel are reared in communes without intense parental involvement. Youths limited to peer group attachments are more likely to use drugs in toxic amounts than those who have extra-parental and peer group involvements. They cannot develop a firm sense of their own identity and, therefore, fail to make satisfactory sexual relationships, complicated by drugs and decreased sexual impulse. Everyone has unconscious feelings, thoughts and problems that vary not only in intensity but in their manifestations, in their degree of localization to one area of the personality and in the amount of incapacity induced. Clearly, adolescents who have an inability to function in any realm need professional help. Those who are in emotional distress but are not incapacitated and those who are incapacitated only in a non-essential area can often continue to function as students or workers and to improve their adjustment to life without help. Youth has great resiliency for many with marked emotional problems seem to emerge from them. The adolescent's own strength of character and his ability to bring to awareness certain of his unconscious conflicts allow him to handle the problems more adequately by repression, suppression, rationalization, sublimation or other process. What is significant is that many such adolescents improve by themselves.

Emotional Reserves

The road to psychological maturity is twisting, hilly and rough, an endless path. Approaching maturity without ever reaching the goal is prophetic; youth beholds the promised land but never realizes it. Some confuse psychological maturation with growth and others with imitation, the basis of the ancient concept of personality. An oak tree begins with an acorn, becomes a seedling, a sapling, a tree. A decade after germination of the acorn the oak has reached maturity; during the next few centuries it will continue to grow in size but it will never be more a tree than it was at ten. Similarly, the human being begins as a fertilized egg, becomes a fetus, an infant, and continues through childhood and adolescence to reach physical maturity at age fifteen years, and then gains experience and wisdom. He will never be more mature in the physical sense than he was at fifteen years but can progress to psychological maturation. Some people are in a state of permanent maturation with slow, delayed psychological growth that ends in death before psychological maturity has been reached. Others are either conformers or rebels ever in a state of zero psychological growth. But, it is possible for the human being to achieve psychological maturity if he works at it. Within a decade after physical maturation, he will continue to grow psychologically and age physically; he will continue to experience the new, to learn to change, to expand his horizons, to grow in judgment and in wisdom; he will become increasingly more alert, more interested, more curious, more universal; he will become more humble, saying "I know" less often than "I hope"; he will grow in psychological stature but will be no more mature psychologically than he was at twenty-five years.

Psychological maturity begins when a person knows who and what he really is as opposed to what he is supposed to be. The eternal maturer is still trying to unravel his own ideas in later years; the conformer is satisfied to act out what he is supposed to be; and the rebel content to refute it. But, the psychologically mature person knows who he is at twenty-five years. He knows who he is at fifty years and he still knows who he is at seventy-five years. He has a sense of sameness, the continuity of basic identity which remains constant despite the passage of time, the variety of experience, the growing accumulation of wisdom. The perennial maturer is steeped in his central core, the eternal question of who am I? His life is dedicated to an unending search for the answer. The conformer has nothing more than his dependence upon the social context in which he is forever stuck like a raisin in a rice pudding. His life is dedicated to maintaining the status quo, to preserving relationship between raisin and rice; and the rebel, somewhat like the conformer, has nothing more than his dependence upon the social context. Where the conformer remains passive and content, the rebel struggles and fights but neither transcends the status quo.

Let us compare the way the world appears to each of these groups: to the psychologically mature person, the world comes alive and constitutes a field in which he lives his life and with which he himself is in constant interaction. He is always aware of his world as he is aware of himself; his world is broad and varied, beautiful and ugly, with love and hate, his to enjoy and his to improve. To him, the world and the self are equally real, equally identifiable, equally meaningful. To the conformer, the world is a gluttonous mass containing the exemplars of the roles he plays and the proponents of the views he parrots. The same world exists for the rebel who fights and resists. Neither the conformer nor the rebel really exists in his own eyes, in his own right. The world exists, authority exists, but his appraisal of himself comes to him only by reflection in the eyes of others. Finally, for the perennial maturer, the world is not much more than a state in which he carries out his ceaseless search for his own identity. He really has little to do with the world, for his energies are turned inward in his own eyes; he and his world are peripheral and irrelevant.

Psychological maturity can be won. The adolescent can find within himself psychological normality. He can lift himself by his own boot-straps above the mediocre average and he can do it systematically with good mind. Youth tends to confuse the mass with the normal, assuming that only the giant can perform with excellence. Who builds on the mob builds on sand. Actually, there are a few great lovers and the rest of us; there are a few great fighters and the rest of us; few great workers and the rest of us; few great artists and the rest of us; few great doctors and the rest of us. In a similar vein, youth assumes that only the giant can think, which is utter nonsense. Every community is reversed out of the unknown ranks and not out of the ranks of those already famous and powerful. Youth must admit to himself that there is procedure for human beings, not just for the gods; he must stick to the path of reasonableness rather than fog, of passion, pride and prejudice to thread his way through a thicket of likes and dislikes, callow enthusiasm, dubious authorities; he must think to grow psychologically.

REFERENCES

Aller, L. P. Jr.: Emotional problems of adolescents. *Northwest Med., 64:* 750-754, 1965.
Ames, L. B. *et al.: Adolescent Rorschach Responses.* New York, Brunner-Mazel, 1971.
Blaine, G. B.: *et al.: Emotional Problems of the Student.* New York, Appleton-Century-Crofts, 1971.
Brown, J. S.: *The Motivation of Behavior.* New York, McGraw-Hill, 1961.

Buhler, C.: The course of human life as a psychological problem. *Hum. Dev., 11*:184-200, 1968.

Dean, D. G.: Can emotional maturity be measured? *Psychol. Rep., 20*:60, 1967.

English, O. S. *et al.: Emotional Problems of Living.* New York, Norton, 1955.

Erikson, E. H.: The problem of ego identity. *J. Am. Psychoanal. Assoc., 4*: 56, 1956.

Eron, L. D.: *The Classification of Behavior Disorders.* Chicago, Aldine, 1966.

Gallagher, J. R.: *Emotional Problems of Adolescents.* New York, Oxford University Press, 1958.

Garrison, A. *et al.: The Psychology of Childhood.* London, Staple, 1967.

Glasser, K.: Emotional problems of adolescence. *Md. State Med. J., 18*:51-4, 1969.

Kagan, J.: Impulsive and reflective children. In J. Krumboltz (Ed.): *Learning and the Educational Process.* Chicago, Rand McNally, 1965.

Kaplan, A.: Philosophical discussion of normality. *Gen. Psychiatry,* Vol. 17, 1967.

Kellner, R. *et al.:* Symptom rating test scores in neurotics and normals. *Br. J. Psychiatry, 113*:525-6, 1967.

Kuhlen, R. G.: *The Psychology of Adolescent Development.* New York, Harper, 1952.

Kurland, H. D. *et al.:* Emotional evaluation of medical patients. *Arch. Gen. Psychiatry, 19*:72-8, 1968.

Monroe, R. R.: *Episodic Behavioral Disorders.* Cambridge, University Press, 1970.

Mowbry, R. M. *et al.: Psychology in Relation to Medicine.* Edinburgh, Livingstone, 1970.

Munn, N. L.: *The Evolution and Growth of Human Behavior.* London, Harrap, 1965.

Piaget, I. *et al.: The Psychology of the Child.* London, Routledge and Kegan Paul, 1969.

Rutter, M.: Psychological development. *J. Child Psychiatry, 11*:49, 1970.

Sarason, S. *et al.:* Psychological and cultural problems in mental subnormality. *Genet. Psychol. Monogr., 57*:3, 1958.

Saul, L. J. *et al.:* The concept of emotional immaturity. *Compr. Psychiatry, 6*:1, 1965.

Scanlon, J. P.: Emotional aspects of youth fitness. *Med. Ann. D.C., 31*:8, 1962.

Sheldon, W. H. *et al.: The Varieties of Temperament. A Psychology of Constitutional Differences.* New York, Harper, 1942.

Silber, E. *et al.:* Adaptive behavior in competent adolescents. *Arch. Gen. Psychiatry, 5*:62, 1961.

Simmons, J. A.: Emotional problems in mental retardation. *Pediatr. Clin. North Am., 15*:957, 1968.

Snyder, R. T.: Personality adjustment, self attitudes, and anxiety differences in retarded adolescents. *Am. J. Ment. Defic., 71*:33-41, 1966.

Stafford-Clark, D.: Drug dependence. *Guy's Hospital Gazette, 83*:298-305, 1969.

Stamell, B. B.: Emotional growth in the adolescent. *Med. Times,* Vol. 92, 1964.

Wallinga, J. V.: The adolescent emotional quandary. *Lancet,* 1962.

CHAPTER V

SOCIAL IMMATURITY

A young Apollo, long-haired,
  Stands dreaming on the verge of strife,
Magnificently unprepared
  For the long littleness of life.

Man evolved as a social animal but less social than some insects. Human sociality is self-awareness manifested by symbolic communication, while insect sociality is inherited instinct. Relating to others is as basic as respiration, circulation, locomotion and metabolism, for man can neither develop normally nor function successfully without other human beings. Thus, isolation, crowding or challenge creates effects of ancient origin unsuitable to current conditions. The humaneness of man is not innate, but a product of group socialization whose norms are transmitted from generation to generation. Each individual incorporates into his life organization the beliefs, ideas and language of the groups to which he belongs. He develops a set of social norms as he develops a social environment. Individuals thus see the world around them not with their eyes alone, for if they did they would all see the same things, but rather through their cultural experiences. Youth needs time to be by himself to discover himself. Such solitude vivifies while isolation kills. It is in solitude that the works of hand, heart and mind are conceived and in solitude that individuality must be affirmed. Yet, the individual who tries to live alone will not succeed as a human being; his heart withers if it does not answer another heart; his mind shrinks if he hears only the echoes of his own thoughts and finds no other inspiration.

Lack of Psychosocial Nutrition

The environment created by man rather than the environment of nature is shifting physical disease to social illness. Disease and disability derive not only from man's constitution and the

151

environment in which he lives but also from his psychologic and behavioral interactions in his social world. It is a deep-seated craving for response from his social environment as fundamental as for food, air and water. Human beings require adequate and balanced amounts of psychosocial provisions, i.e. attention, affection, approval, guidance, care, protection, sacrifice—all love components. Any deficiency in these social nutrients may produce psychosocial malnutrition—deprivation when the social provisions are inadequate; intoxication, when overabundant; and injury when either deprivation or intoxication become poisonous, despite the human ability to adjust within limits to variations in modes of providing such abstract supplies.

Children reared under primitive conditions participating in the economy behave in an altruistic way as recipients of psychosocial nutrition, while those in class or caste systems, nonparticipating in community work, behave in an egotistic manner as nonrecipients in psychosocial nutrition. Adolescents reveal sociobehavioral and physical disorders with equal frequency and intensity or both disorders may coexist. And correction of the biosocial features of any illness will accelerate recovery of physical illness. Indeed, there is no physical illness without psychosocial illness and vice versa. When man is sick, he is sick all over. It takes psychosocial nutrients to raise the ailing spirit of another human in the innermost core of his being. The transcendental force of love thus inverts human behavior of sensibility to trifles and insensibility to other beings.

Psychosocial provision is a positive encounter with another human being on the basis of love and sensibility. It penetrates the psychic wall that separates one individual from another. The transcendent power of love vitalizes the other being via a common bond and feeling and the understanding embodied in coexistence. The Greeks called it agape or devotion; Buber, "we"; existentialists, "sorge" or care of another person. To be creative in human relationships is to open oneself freely to the wants and needs of another being and to take into one's self the other person's being unconditionally. What one gives to another and receives from him is himself as a whole being.

Youth needs two kinds of love—unselfish love for the being of another person and/or selfish love or deficiency love. The former is welcomed into consciousness and is completely enjoyed. It can never be sated and grows in content and intensity to mystic heights with a minimum of anxiety-hostility. The two beings are independent of each other, more autonomous, less jealous, less needful but simultaneously more eager to help the other toward self-actualization; they become more altruistic, generous and fostering. It is both a cognitive and emotional reaction; it creates the partner and confers a self-image, a feeling of love-worthiness and respect. Worthiness which stimulates growth for nonlove is nonconducive to growth or maturation. Deficiency love, on the other hand, is at a lower level, less valuable subjective experience for both donor and recipient. There is gratification without the love-worthiness of true love. It is impossible to love a second time what youth has really ceased to love. It is superficial, synthetic, satisfying without glorifying the partner in a transcended bond of deep-seated devotion.

Love does not fractionate and partition; it unites and builds. Love does not reduce the other being to something else, but with reverence accepts him as is. Love is not blind, but insightful. It is the summum bonum of care, responsibility, faith and sacrifice. Care is total concern for another individual's well-being via consummate love and productive anxiety. It embraces love and sensibility, and hate and indifference; it can be creative or neurotic. The parent who cares for his child is anxiously concerned for him, but his anxiety makes for a sense of viability. Life takes on an inner delight because one knows that in caring for the other, one gives oneself to him without asking anything in return. It transcends the separation that our uniqueness engenders to effect a union with each other. Love and care are means for the liberation of the human spirit not for its enslavement. Love is the creator of the community.

Responsibility is a detachable burden easily shifted to the shoulders of God, Fate, Fortune, Luck. To be a man is precisely to be responsible. In the darkness of night, the parent rises to minister to the sick child because he is a life for which she deeply cares. Compassion provokes action with no thought of where the moral responsibility lies. Care cannot be rationalized for it is primary and unconditional; the spontaneous engagement of one life is the life of another. Care is intrinsic; responsibility, extrinsic regard for the well-being of another person. Responsibility is care rationalized. Man is what he loves. In loving another, he is that other, and other is himself.

Sacrifice is selfless devotion of one person to another. Sacrificial love is a giving, not an asking encounter; it is unconditional; it depends on its own power to fulfill the being of the other. It is a love in which self-love is suppressed by selflessness, in constant need of a reassuring faith. Sacrificial love means self-renunciation and commitment to another individual. One feels most alive when one cares or sacrifices for another. When the sacrifice is mutual, one person is able to understand the other in the depth of his being. Each comprehends the other mystically rather than rationally. Love reveals the secret of the other being and each transcends his aloneness. All psychological nutrients—attention, affection, approval, guidance, care, protection, responsibility—are dynamic components of love that depend on faith for fulfillment. Faith is the unconditional belief in the sanctity and trust of one human being for another.

The adolescent craves psychosocial nutrients for cultivation of the self as of the body. He is imbued with the spirit of the time but must have meaningful ties to parents, people, ideas and symbols derived from the past and projecting into the future. This inner bond gives him a sense of transcendence from the material "machine" upkeep to the abstract "self" maturation to create a sense of immortality. Displacement of psychosocial forces by counterfeit nurturance leads to the development of immature personalities, youth rebellions, rote behavior, pseudoattachments and emotional disorders. This psychosocial deficiency can be corrected by adhering to the good life with our last muscle—the heart. It is the heart always that sees, before the head can see. And woman is the most sensitive, the must susceptible, the best index of the coming day. It takes feminine knowing to fulfill this biologic obligation to children and then to youth like the goddess

Demeter who taught mankind to raise itself above beasts and become the giver of immortality.

Lack of Social Sense

The earth is a beehive—all enter by the same door but live in different cells. Some solitary wretches leave the rest of mankind, only as Eve left Adam, to meet the devil in private. Then isolation becomes the mother of existence. Failure of the young to express needs blocks the very inception of socialization. The ghastly doughy child becomes deprived, malnourished, autistic, inhuman. Social isolation of feral children presents a complete picture of such an asocial existence, running on all fours, resisting all efforts to teach them to walk upright, absence of any form of language other than a variety of vocal sounds, mimicking animals in whose vicinity they have lived; emotional explosions reflecting anger and fear, absence of cleanliness or modesty, absence of any pattern of eating and behavior. A social animal has many advantages. The parent teaches the child, the craftsman teaches his apprentice. Useful behavior is acquired under social contingencies and verbal behavior from social interactions. The child becomes both a speaker and a listener in possession of a repertoire applied by himself for self-knowledge. Deprived of a social environment, a human being remains feral, without verbal behavior, without self-awareness as a person, without techniques of self-management, without skills to grow, develop and mature.

Man is barely human in his behavior exposed to diversity of social and cultural patterns, yet certain behavior constants bear testimony to basic biologic attributes: language, cooperative labor, courtship patterns, codes of family life, care of the young, fire-making, cooking, dancing, incest, taboos, gift-giving, superstitions, belief in magic, status differentiation, religious rituals and funeral rites. In some cultures attitudes towards children are warm and accepting with all adult members of a particular endogenous group providing care and feeding for them, while in others only the barest essentials of child care are given grudgingly. The mother remains the particular caretaker of the child in most societies while the father controls emotional relationships. In some groups children are subjected to severe abuse with subsequent abandonment, infanticide, and cannibalism during food shortages. Clearly, the characteristics considered basic human attributes vary with the function of social structures and the hazards posed by survival.

Society plays a structuring role in the life of the adolescent from primitive rites and rituals to organized systems of apprenticeships. He feels insecure when his society is in unrest and danger yet must learn to live in the face of rapid social change with uncertainty and ambiguity. There are no adequate models of identification as society becomes more complex without immediate solutions to adolescent problems. And so some teen-agers demur and seek relevance in social action, while others create a simpler society to themselves with peer groups. Adolescent life then becomes a matter of priorities rather than real interaction with society.

How does social sense develop? It begins as primary socialization by interaction with personal attachment to members of the family. It is the first condition of social happiness—the sense of a common life. It constitutes a society of a certain number of individuals living in a particular way in a particular place at a particular time—nothing else. It gradually inculcates morality, love, friendship and justice from its adults expressing mutual aid to its constituents, even though these essential qualities of social life are so intangible. Each society develops and progresses only on the condition that it obeys these fundamental laws, otherwise it perishes. A child considers social existence as good if it makes for physical and spiritual health; and bad if it hurts, dwarfs and distorts life.

The happiness of a child's life is made up of minute fractions— a kiss, a smile, a kind look, a pat, heartfelt praise, and countless infinitesimals of genial feelings, but the supreme happiness is the feeling that he is loved. Which child has not his desire? Or, having it, is satisfied? If not, he chooses a friendless existence, becomes lonely, and develops a solicitude for things, and his relation to them begins to become love, and lays him open to pain. Once the lonely child remains distinct from his group, he offers his hand to whomever he encounters. He relates in parallel rather than perpendicular manner and acts like a loner until secondary socialization brings choice individuals into his selective social milieu. He will love others in much the same way that others love him. He will incorporate in his personality much that prevails in his social setting. If it be loving, he tends to be loving and his obligations to others become closely bound to his obligations to himself. It is to the credit of the human family that it loves more readily than it hates, the one tenet of nature that can make the whole world kin.

The school child gives something to others as an integral part of his need to be protected and loved and gives himself to enterprises in which he joins others. But failure in early socialization is evidenced by selfishness, compensatoriness, and/or aggressiveness, yet the outcome of his struggle with his own antisocial impulses leads to idealistic actions. To master his own impulses, he strives for a kind of perfection and sets for himself high goals of moral achievement which are accompanied by high expectations of other people. He becomes absorbed in the discovery, exploration and mastery of himself as a social being. He discovers inner rudiments of compassion and assertiveness, of cooperation and competition. He develops friends and enemies and learns techniques for dealing with both effectively. He evolves a culture of his own, enabling the cultivation of social attributes without adult interference. He wants to be part of the childhood group, within it, not on top of it as a winner, despite parental urgings. He gradually learns to behave socially by direct personal association with others who have been acculturated in the social system. He thus acquires the knowledge provided by the particular society's culture according to his ways of participating in the social system. But the socially immature youth is deficient as an effective participant ever remaining a lonely spectator of his society.

The adolescent begins to shift his attachments from the family to outsiders. He likes to lose himself in a group, to be fully accepted by it, to remain uncritically loyal to it, and to be indiscriminately hostile to outside groups that threaten its existence. With several in the group there is something bold in the air; direct things get said which would frighten two people alone so conscious of each inch of their nearness to one another. They feel safe in a group; they not only talk together but do things together. The young are faithful to individuals of their choice; the older grow more loyal to situations and to types. At this formative stage, ideas of right and wrong are based on the thinking of the group, particularly of its leaders. Each member likes to perform hard tasks in the interest of the group and be rewarded by it for whatever he does. Unquestioning loyalty to the group becomes generalized to larger social units such as the school, city, state and nation unless challenged by fundamental weaknesses in the makeup of these institutions.

Uncritical devotion to any group is a low order of responsibility for it does not require much ego development, education or intelligence. Moreover, it is likely to be short-lived, dissolving when the group dissolves because it constantly has to be nourished by group influence. Youth goes through this stage and emerges from it learning not only to work with others but also to be wary of blind loyalty or uncritical rejection of other groups. The youngster who misses this stage in early adolescence must have another chance to go through it later. It applies especially to the aesthetic boy who never could keep up with the group and so comes home to his mother and his homework. When he arrives at college he rejects sports, remains the intellectual, bars social feelings, and becomes alienated from society. Every adolescent needs the experience of group loyalty followed by the chance to criticize the group and compare it with others to avoid alienation and compulsion to do one's duty. All comparisons are odious; they will disenchant him with his college, his community, his nation. He will complain of hypocrisy and criticize adults' failings while his own values are challenged by exposure to other cultures and to new experiences. Some adolescents resolve the conflicts created by disenchantment; others discover that there are goals that can be accepted after critical examination; and the pursuit of these goals may well serve the basic needs of personality. They will find great satisfaction in socially valuable work for a whole range of inner needs. Socially responsible behavior can become a channel through which even childish needs can be expressed by an adolescent personality.

The immature adolescent does what authority says rather than what he himself has thought best. He is not in a position to take responsible action on the larger social front because he lacks self-confidence and has uncertain views of what he can do. He is preoccupied with his own problems, with his inner self. Our current high pressure system entails problems of self-preservation, of survival. It isn't important to come out on top in his group. What matters is to be the one who comes out alive in the struggle. The college stay means capitulating to voluntary servitude to expand the intellect, the feelings and the physique to emerge into an integrated personality. Once he is aroused by social and political issues he needs not only the support of a sympathetic group but confidence in his own decision-making, a confidence born only of experience. Nevertheless, the immature adolescent fails to develop a sense of social responsibility; he lacks the initiative to catalyze social relationships essential for maturation. He suffers not only from ignorance of the world at large but from lack of opportunity to be of service. He passes up chances to be helpful and loses self-content in competing successfully with others. As this feeling continues, the self builds up to seek opportunities to sacrifice in some action of great significance. The only cure for self-content is an actual experience of being helpful to others in a radically different setting.

An adolescent needs this experience to test the adequacy of his judgment, to familiarize him with what he can do, and above all to learn about the self-fulfillment of being of service to others. Society is a kind of parent to its members. If both are to thrive its values must be clear, coherent and acceptable. But we live in a commercial society whose adolescents, indifferent to social ritual, must be provided with blueprints and specifications for evoking the right tone at every occasion. To be in society may be a bore to youth, but to be out of it, a tragedy. He remains a loner, cooperates with others, develops recreational interests with others but favors no stable friendships and remains dependent upon his home and parents. He scores low on the Vineland Social Maturity Scale, a measure of the development of self-reliance.

Lack of Social Values

The child's basic social and emotional needs are at the core of an equilibrium-seeking system that adapts through growth and experience. Its mechanism is distinct from cognitive adaptation. The social stages depict successive states that offer useful, heuristic landmarks of maturation. Society expects certain accomplishments, certain competence and certain behaviors from humans at certain ages. There is a time for this or that kind of self-discipline, a time for legal responsibility and so on. The social expectations are formal, embedded in codes of law, and the church and the school; they are informally embedded in many ways in which people affirm their expectations about other people. These social mores are dynamic factors in development, designed to bring the expectations of society into phase with the development of youth, exerting all kinds of demand upon him. Society expects him to show self-discipline, human understanding, resourcefulness, personal initiative, responsibility. The patterning of social behavior is determined by development of propriate traits of personal value schemata. Without values there would be no socialization, and without socialization, values would not exist; and personal values are derived from public values. The child internalizes parents' values and so they become his own; once internalized the values are deemed highly personal and constitute the perceptual self. They provide orientation for interpersonal relationships within the family and society on the compass which provides the sense of direction in the maze of social relations throughout life. Mature values are gradually acquired in group living during puberty. The leader of the clique influences the adolescent most when loyalties are split between parents and peers, but the family still remains the prime source of interpersonal standards.

The life values of the adolescent compared with those of his parents are no longer determined by authoritative right and wrong but by abstract reasoning that leads to mature judgment. Moral values for the child are adjudged by his parents; for the pre-adolescent, by his peer group; for the adolescent, by his perceptual self. Youth must decide how he is valuable in society rather than how valuable he is at home. He is no longer a creature concerned with the present for he must learn from the past and plan for the future to acquire value schemata as the propriate behavior. Values cannot be changed suddenly, else loss of continuity of the perceptual self leads to disorientation, anxiety and depression producing loneliness, moodiness, and lack of direction. The core of conflict reflects identity integration vs. identity diffusion. A stable sense of identity involves three deep-seated changes: external sanctions give way to internal; experiences of prohibition give way to preferences; habits of obedience give way to self-guidance.

The maintenance of home values established for a personal way of life soon comes into conflict with world social values of material success. The greater the disparity between what the child has been led to expect and what the adolescent perceives as accepted values, the greater the internal conflict. As a rule, youth adopts a dual set of values—one for his peers and one for the world. Such a schism creates internal instability. He never knows his current—AC or DC. Youth's value schemata provide half of our new dictionary terms of adolescent slang and the other half comes from scientific terminology. The late adolescent's ultimate goal is acceptance into an adult group. He needs to adopt society's values to guide him along that path. Unfortunately, the mores of western society are undergoing such continuous changes as to make such adolescent planning impossible. Youth's dilemma is further complicated by mass media considering the adolescent as big business. They accentuate his unique role as a separate component of society for profit, an isolation that creates endless adolescence devoid of independent action and/or creating a personal philosophy of life.

Lack of Personal Identity

Adolescence begins with sudden but subtle changes in personality and ends with slow but imperceptible changes in maturity within two or three years. But in the immature adolescent, both transitions at onset and termination are difficult to delineate because of pronounced distinctive features of normal adolescence. All emotions are feebler than those of the average youth with none of the rapid fluctuation of feeling; none of the depth of love or hate; none of the interest or boredom; none of the daydreams or yearnings for gratification; and, none of the violent urges to experience new emotions. He prefers quiescence rather than activity, routine rather than surprise. His failure of self-criticism parallels the failure of reality testing and persists with failure to perceive incongruities in himself. He is totally unaware of the world about him; it is not selfishness nor self-centeredness but inability to concern himself with persons and events that do not impinge upon him personally.

The adolescent's main task in life is to give birth to himself. He is confronted with a new interpersonal dimension with a sense of ego identity at the positive end and a sense of role confusion at the negative end. The primary task is to bring together all of the things he has learned about himself as a child, student, athlete, friend, scout and integrate the diverse images of himself into a composite whole for continuity with the past in preparation for the future. The young person who succeeds in this endeavor develops a sense of psychosocial identity, a sense of who he is, who he has been and where he is going. The immature adolescent, however, does not attain this level of personality crystallization, remains in a state of confusion about his being, and enters the final stage of development with mistrust, doubt, guilt and inferiority.

The sense of personal identity not only depends upon developmental processes but upon the social milieu. The young man who sees traditional values broken down by technological advances finds it difficult to reconcile his home upbringing with world standards. He seeks causes to give his life meaning and direction and joins youth groups in the new activities. The girl reared as a secondary citizen at home finds difficulty in achieving a sense of psychosocial identity and remains confused, though relatively mature for her developmental age. To be nobody but yourself in a world which is doing its best, night and day, to make you everybody else means to fight the hardest battle which any human being can fight. Our culture impedes the delineation of any faithful self-image, indeed of any clear image whatever. We do not break images; there are few iconoclasts among us; instead, we blur and soften them.

Role confusion is the negative sense of not knowing what you are, where you belong or to whom you belong. It abounds in all young persons who cannot attain a positive sense of personal identity either because of an unfortunate childhood or difficult social circumstances. Such confusion predominates in the delinquents, the promiscuous and the revolutionary. Indeed, some adolescents seek a negative identity opposite to the one prescribed for them by their family to be lauded by their peers who can alienate them from society. Even negative identity may be preferable to no identity at all. A strong sense of identity, positive or negative, gives the adolescent the idea he can do no wrong; too little accomplishes the same. Yet failure to establish a clear sense of identity during adolescence does not lead to perpetual failure. And, the one who attains a sense of working ego identity at adolescence will necessarily encounter threats to that identity as he goes through life.

Confronting problems at one stage in life is no guarantee against the reappearance of these problems in later stages or of ever finding new solutions to them. Youth wanders rather than migrates, but in the end there is always a certain peace in being what one is, in being that completely. Even the condemned youth feels that joy. All psychosocial development is an individual step-by-step ego identification process initiated by maternal identification. He conceives himself as the same through time with sameness for all others. This creates an identity crisis from puberal changes and conflicting expectations of him in a pluralistic society, complicated by the need to make final choices about the opposite sex and a vocation. It is characterized by deficiency feelings of the life stuff needed to get started as an independent citizen; it threatens an identity diffusion in our society where the adolescent status is ambiguous, expectations ill-defined, and mutual evaluations distorted.

Resolution of the identity crisis is in the fate of peer relations under the motto: "Resolve to be thyself, and know that he who finds himself loses his misery." Adolescents offer one another feedback by stereotyping behavior in their private groups. It enables youth to experiment with patterns of love and living amongst friends to evolve the optimal style of life based on an acceptable identity. All the ramifications of personality are tested in fads and fancies of raiment, transformations of appearance, manner of dating, sensuousness of love affairs, types of socialization, moods, and exhilarations—all components of the central developmental task of molding the self. Failure to develop a personal identity leads to a breakdown that may be manifest as depression, acute anxiety, hysteria, psychosomatic illness, confusion, disorientation, aggression, delinquent behavior, anorexia nervosa, or drug addiction.

Social functioning is the resultant of biological equipment, early training, everyday experience and environmental forces. Most important is the sociofamilial environment in which the youth is reared, the setting in which he observes how others behave, and the values their culture maintains. The environment's responses are determined by forces beyond his control—sex, appearance, interest and behavior that prevail in his family. There are critical periods during which social skills are learned best; the more an individual is emotionally aroused during such a learning period the more likely he will master it. Once the period is past, the likelihood of his acquiring the skill will diminish. But youth may not learn to socialize because he is ostracized; another may fumble socially because seizures disrupt participation; still another may be backward. Home training can compensate for social deficiencies as illustrated by two Mongol adolescents, one the son of a peddler who behaved like a wild animal in the waiting room and the other the son of a college president who behaved like a diplomat.

What are the minimum standards of good social functioning? Actions speak louder than words; but we must consider the words and/or feelings accompanying them in all possible social relationships. The action patterns are assessed from the standpoint of energy level, vigor, adroitness, directness and effectiveness. We are just as interested in what the adolescent does as in what he does not do. In his relations to people, he has established various patterns of social encounter—major attachments and minor devotions, best friends and worst enemies. We must study the quality, depth, consistency and satisfactions of the linkages, the kinds of ambivalence betrayed, the active and passive dependencies exhibited. Development of full social responsibility requires experience in social action helpful to others; it tests adequacy of adolescent judgment, familiarizes him with the limits of his ability, teaches him the self-fulfillment that comes from being of service to others, the binding effect of serving a friend and the befriending effect of serving an enemy. The patterns of the adolescent social integration are reflected in the way he works and in the way he plays—too much or too little produces a gross imbalance in his life style. Each individual must find satisfactions in his life efforts—food, warmth, sexual relations, peer activities, chosen endeavors and creative hobbies. All will be colored by intangibles that dominate the course of his life—personal concerns and social considerations, ideals and aspirations, attitudes and responsibilities, prejudices and predilections, self-image and self-confidence, religious feelings and growing philosophy of life. It takes longitudinal evaluation of an adolescent's life to assess his social competence.

Youth faces new social expectations in heterosexual relations in context with a peer group after preadolescent socialization with the same sex clique. Such togetherness is a substitute sense of community, a counterfeit communion. From time to time it becomes clear that youth begins to appreciate, even respect a group of peers gathered in a room, each of whom taken by himself, he may consider of no account. The profoundest affinities are those most readily felt. Yet the increasingly intense heterosexual association is neither initiated nor pursued on an individual basis. And the extent of peer contact is no direct function of the actual number of acquaintances. Both experiences with the sexes, singly and collectively, lay the foundation for organizing social activities in the neighborhood, social environment of the peer group in the same socioeconomic status formed. The highest and lowest ranking positions stabilize first while the middle positions are filled more slowly. The levellers level down as far as themselves but cannot bear levelling up to themselves. Community cliques are part of a hierarchy with leaders for each group and the whole organization. The leader sets the pace of social development while the social center relieves the tension created by the pressure for achieving heterosexuality. In the crowd, a mass mind operates—a mind without subtlety, a mind without compassion, a mind uncivilized.

Conformity is the theme of the swan song to gain and maintain group status even though every new adjustment is a crisis in self-esteem. Actually, there are no conditions to which youth cannot become accustomed, especially if he sees that all those around him live in the same way. Adapt or perish is the inexorable imperative of the group. This presents youth with ideas and values at a time when he is organizing and stabilizing his own system of values and goals. To him there is one quality more important than know-how, i.e. know-what to determine not only how to accomplish his goal, but what his goal should be. And a good peer culture offers such life objectives in a suitable setting for evaluation and incorporation. The talking period between eleven and thirteen gives way to the doing period between nineteen and twenty-one.

Lack of Social Adaptation

Society could never be run by adolescents because social organization requires its members to replace self-interest with real interest in others. In all authoritarian societies, the status of the majority of the people resembles that of children more than that of adults. The rulers take care of their subjects who express their maturity by taking care of their progeny. All social manifestations of productivity are absent in contrast to the free societies in ancient Greece and in western civilization which were prolific in artistic, literary and scientific productivity. Democracy releases the energies of every human being. The adolescent will learn to assume responsibility for his own activities if his self-control is not based on fear of external authorities. It must be rooted in his own conscience that develops through positive identification with adults. But if the socialization is achieved primarily through fear of punishment, only a grudging type of conformity will develop. Social behavior is continuous rather than discrete. Its manifestations reflect a composite of traits such as intelligence, introversion, emotionality and sociality which vary from high to low or from strong to weak. All behavior is complex since any trait can be dissociated into an unlimited number of components. Together, these three dimensions—basic temperament, affective relations and instinctive patterns—constitute personality which is both situational and transitional, specific and nonspecific.

The socially maturing adolescent gradually progresses in several areas—acceptance of one's self by innate adjustment of his appearance and his ability; acceptance of one's self in relation to a group by recognizing the variability of one's status and the specificity of leadership; acceptance of others in spite of their differences and the unpredictability of their behavior; acceptance of others in relation to one's self with the relativity of friendship, and the means by which one may make one's self acceptable to others. Successful adjustments form the background against which all other activities are judged. Indeed, all other forms of learning assume secondary importance. Learning to adjust to the realities of one's own endowment and one's relationship to others is most effective in a heterosexual group; hence the universal justification of coeducation in normal family fashion from birth to exitus. Such a free school atmosphere provides a greater degree of mental health and a better transition to the acceptance of adult status with mature responsibility.

The adolescents' life will be successful if the power of their accommodation is equal to the necessary and sufficient adjustment of internal and external changes. We can promote vigorous social adaptation balanced in its concern for self, family and community, and responsible for future social planning, by providing adolescents with acceptable continuity of affection, guidance and protection. We must provide them with approved levels of stimulation that respect their individual and collective tolerance with opportunities for social experiments. We must enable them to live their independent lives in a humane community rather than to be lived by drives or submerged by society. Otherwise, neurosis becomes the great saboteur; it undermines youth's health, destroys schooling, diminishes working efficiency, ruins social development, complicates peer relations, engenders hostilities towards fellowman. At every level, emotional problems intrude on effective living. Physical needs, ego status and social requirements are vitiated, leading to collapse in adaptation. The capacity to mediate stress, to gratify essential needs, to endure deprivation, to deal with conflicts constructively are all insured by an harmonious blending of the various facets of personality. It is through the operation of the personality that youth manages functions in society. A balanced personality makes for an adequate adjustment; an unbalanced personality engenders maladjustments.

The unbalanced personality emerges from blocks in maturation that may create incomplete reality concepts, imperfect social control over bodily functions, diminished assertiveness, inadequate sexual function, improper mastery of hostile impulses, deficient group identification, faulty integration of social values and impaired acceptance of the social role. All aberrant behavior patterns reveal conflicts, stress and anxiety and the common denominator of the neurotic personality. They are not in themselves pathological, nor are the coping attempts of adjusting, for each may be utilized constructively. A rock in one's path may be a stumbling block or a building block according to the caliber of maturation. Social maturing involves an inevitable clash between inner needs and reality demands, between innate drives and restricted acculturation. Compromises are inevitable either by gratification of needs by socially condoned practices or by sublimation, displacement, transformation, renunciation and repression. Successful adaptation presupposes not absence of conflict but its reasonable solution consistent with what is best for the adolescent at the time of its mediation. Modulation of strivings from the unconscious, of immediate conscious ego needs, of ethical and moral values, and of environmental standards is the essence of good adjustment, all anchored in reality. All adjustment aims necessitate a flexibility of defenses, an ability to shift from one set of maneuvers to another, conditioning existing needs and prevailing exigencies to his own life and the life of others.

Adolescence presents both continuity and change. The same major developmental tasks of finding one's self, of gaining a secure place in society and of achieving a set of moral values to live by remain for this as for all preceding generations the fundamental challenges which have to be met and mastered. Failure at each of these tasks can result in serious social and psychological maladjustments. Adult help is mandatory, both in the form of parental concern and sympathetic guidance and in extreme cases of social misfits and educational dropouts at the level of preventive community action. The future belongs to youth, hence the traditional aspect of the adolescent role as the shaper of culture presents increased urgency in a fast-moving world to be dominated by cybernetics and automation and challenged by space travel while poverty and starvation remain unsolved. At the same time there are drastic changes in outlook and behavior on the part of youth. It is not merely a matter of odd raiment but a more tolerant attitude towards one another, coupled with rejection of paternalism, defiance of authoritarianism, dissatisfaction with political systems, struggle for equal participation in decision-making, fulfillment of which will result in reduction in anxiety by enrichment of the democratic way of life.

Lack of Respect for Society

Society is not only immoral but immortal. It can afford to commit any kind of folly and indulge in any sort of vice; it cannot be destroyed. How can the adolescent reconcile his newly formed ideals—the imaginative understanding of that which is desirable in that which is possible? His body can be mobilized by law but where shall he find that which will help him believe in what he must do, so that he can fight through the transitional period to personal victory? He did not enter society to become worse than he was before, but to have those rights better secured. He wants to develop his own personality, use his own talents before becoming a speck of society's gigantic personality. His rebellion defines his caliber of being in showing no respect for place, person or time.

Morality is acquired, not inborn—it is the custom of one's country and the feeling of one's peers. Every system of morality is a body of imperfect generalizations, expressed in emotional terms—blind obediency to words of command. But without civic morality communities perish; without personal morality their survival has no value. Some children are socialized to tame their impulses to comply with law and order; others, to exercise altruism, compassion for the less fortunate. The important thing is not the moral perfection to which an adolescent attains but the process of attainment. Conceptions of moralization are not a process of internalization of external cultural rules through verbal teaching, punishment or identification. On the contrary, all evidence points to the existence of a series of internally patterned transformation of social concepts and attitudes. Youth's current shift to restore moral conflicts in favor of human ends defies institutional norms via protest, activism and anomie. Yet man is essentially a moral being even when he denies the existence of all morality. That very denial already becomes the foundation of new morality.

The rebel deviate or delinquent acts not out of wickedness but for the satisfaction of an urge, an appetite, a whim. He is a presentist, who styles the present moment an extraordinary crisis and lives for it. The word now is like a bomb through the window. He must act immediately; he cannot relate himself to the past or the future. He finds no *raison d'etre* in life and has no reason to develop any responsibility for his way of life. Our civilization applauds quick action whatever the consequences. Society prepares the crime; the delinquent commits it. And most delinquents commit great crimes because of their scruples about petty ones. The chief problem in any community cursed with juvenile delinquents is not punishment of the deranged youth but the preventing of young from being trained in crime.

Delinquent behavior reaches a peak during adolescence. Psychologically it may be due to deformed ego and superego formation, poor impulse control in organic brain damage, severe deprivation that prompts immediate impulse gratification, neurotic conflict with inadequate sexual identification or strong guilt feelings, family interference, gang association. All adolescents are juvenile delinquents—asocial and amoral—in the laws for traffic, littering, loitering, drinking and drugging. Delinquency is a symptom of unconscious symbolic meaning with multiple causes manifest in impulsive adolescents by pleasure seeking and imaginary thinking that lead to chain reactions and crime. Social psychopathology points to failure of the adolescent to fit into the normal pattern of living and reacting in the framework of his own environment. It indicates the need to look beyond the delinquent act and find the underlying personal causes that compromise the struggle between two opposing wishes: immediate gratification of tension and a conscience that flaunts reality.

The adolescent has not been able to incorporate the inhibitions of the environment because of his immaturity. The misbehaving adolescent may well have been misbehaving from early childhood as a result of disturbances of brain metabolism or brain injury. Early danger signals in feeding, toilet training, bedwetting, fire-setting, running away are followed later by thievery, glue sniffing, sexual offenses, responsive early to psychologic and/or neurological therapy. Despite normal intelligence he often shows lack of judgment, control and inability to foresee the inevitable results of misbehavior. There may be clear-cut neurologic abnormalities indicating brain malfunction or injury that correlates with hyperactivity, explosive behavior and poor control leading to criminal behavior—larceny, arson, mayhem or murder. Some display temper tantrums, unreasonable fears or actual seizures, emanating from bad family background.

Punitive treatment of the initial delinquency reenforces counteraggression. Drug therapy with anticonvulsants, tranquilizers and environmental psychotherapy will rehabilitate half of these misfits. Every effort to provide psychotherapy for youth with antisociality disorders is doomed before it begins. It is almost impossible to modify youth's pathological way of receiving and responding to the social order. He attends a session only because of the pressure exerted by his family or probation officer. He experiences anxiety about his social behavior because the negative social feedback promotes an internalization of the social rules necessary to modify his behavior. But the desire dissipates as soon as his initial discomfort declines. He gradually falls back into the pattern of giving no thought to his past or his future.

SOCIAL MATURATION

Man is foreordained to be a social creature by his reproductive pattern and prolonged dependency. He carries the vestiges of his birth—the slime and eggshells of his primeval past—with him to the end of his days. A man may never become human, remaining frog, lizard, ant; or become human above the waist, fish below. Whatever the animal embodiment of the primitive human, the manifestations reflect such residuum. The fish in the water is silent; the animal on earth is noisy; the bird in the air is singing. And so man has in him the silence of the sea, the noise of the earth, and the music of the air. He is a knot, a web, a mesh unto which his relationships are tied in the daily struggle for survival culminating in social maturity in the making.

Every man is a unit whose human nature is constant, human culture variable and social heritage changing at an alarming rate. There is no continuum of uniform genetic identity but genetic transmission of physical and psychic potentialities and no patterned transmission of social or experimental components, hence the inevitable break between generations. Social heritage can never be frozen; the social environment created by man himself cannot be fixed. In the past, cultural change has been imperceptible within a single generation. Today, the nature of our culture is becoming difficult to identify. There is a social gulf between successive generations despite the great extensions of formal education which ought to have stabilized the social heritage. Society must take steps to slow down the pace of social change to a speed that primitive human nature can tolerate. That will be very difficult to achieve.

Social Maturation Tests and Measurements

Bills, R. *et al.*: An index of adjustment and values. *J. Consult. Psychol.*, 15: 257-261, 1951.

Bowers, P. *et al.*: Developmental correlates of role-playing ability. *Child Dev.*, 30:499-508, 1965.

Crandall, V. C. *et al.*: A children's social desirability questionnaire. *J. Consult. Psychol.*, 29:27-36, 1965.

Cunningham, R.: *Understanding Group Behavior of Boys and Girls.* Teachers College, Columbia University, New York, 1951.

Farber, B. *et al.*: *Family Organization and Parent-child Communications.* Monographs of the Society for Research in Child Development, No. 7, 28, 1963.

Finley, C. B.: The social opinions inventory as a measure of social maturity. *Child Dev.*, 26:81-90, 1955.

Harris, D. B.: A scale for measuring attitudes of social responsibility in children. *J. Abnorm. Soc. Psychol.*, 55:322-326, 1957.

Kantor, M. B.: *Some Consequences of Residential and Social Mobility for Adjustment of Children. Mobility and Mental Health*, Springfield, Thomas, 1965, pp. 86-122.

London, P.: Developmental aspects of discrimination in relation to adjustment. *Genet. Psychol. Monogr.* 57:293-336, 1958.

McReynolds, P. *et al.*: Relation of object curiosity to psychological adjustment in children. *Child Dev.*, 32:393-400, 1961.

Marshall, H. R.: Differences in parent and child reports of the child's experience in the use of money. *J. Educ. Psychol.*, 54:132-317, 1963.

Pintner, R. *et al.*: An adjustment inventory for use in schools for the deaf. *Am. Ann. Deaf*, 82:152-167, 1937.

Sears, R. R. *et al.*: *Patterns of Child-Rearing.* Evanston, Row, Peterson, 1957.

Stott, D. H.: The assessment of mentally handicapped children. *Med. Officer*, 110:235-239, 1963.

Ulmer, R. A. *et al.*: Children's minimal social behavior scale: a short, objective measure of personality functioning (10 year level). *Psychol. Rep.* 22:283-286, 1968.

Social Origins

Social behavior arises from the dependence of every individual on others. No existing form of life is truly solitary and no organism is completely independent of others at all times. The formation of a social bond begins with the approach of one organism to another. The reaction is neutralized by withdrawal, favored by low intensity stimulation, energized by high intensity stimulation. Similar reaction patterns chart the behavioral changes between maturation and experience. The study of social behavior is a study of cooperation between or among individuals with an innate tendency of one to give a signal and the other to respond. The resultant effect of the encounter is determined by the mutuality of the participants. The mutual understanding of the entente leads to cooperative action, and when multiplied in arithmetic or geometric proportions creates socialization. For the adolescent, it is a ceaseless struggle in every personal encounter over the domination of personality development by the innate self, by the people who raise youth, and the society in which youth will participate as an adult member. There is an input process of acquisition determined by what is done to the child and an output resultant in the caliber of the adolescent.

Early socialization involves gradual reduction of behavioral diversities: the child learns to abandon some of the many possible responses he could make to any given situation and to make only the response that is acceptable to the culture in which he develops. The process involves action that changes the response patterns, but the child brings his own array of organismic attributes which monitor the social experiences. He can adapt to a wide range of caretaking patterns, but deviant development appears if a necessary base level of sensory and emotional stimulation is not maintained. The programming of social events cannot be random in order to obtain optimal development, but must correspond to the child's own intrinsic timetable of developmental needs. Social development is greatly influenced by the first events in a child's life, i.e. the first loss of baby teeth, the first degradation from corporal punishment, the first occasion for special situations involving an audience, the first continuous relationship with sympathetic adults other than parents, the first regular deviation from family-regulated toilet behavior, the first significant exposure to community-wide infectious disease hazard, the first sexual experience, the first exploration of hundreds of new experiences.

Social Emergence

Social development is purposeful in unfolding, orderly in integration, progressive in experience. It is determined by parent and sibling relationship in a home atmosphere of personal encounters. The preschooler acquires new skills through play which enables him to relate to his group, to distinguish what is his from that of others and to share agreeably without usurping. The school child clarifies his innate capacities for the social good, relates to others outside the family while challenged by every experience. If pushed beyond his capacity, he develops attitudes of confusion, conflict and frustration. How he emerges from personal relations depends on the soundness of his early development and on the reactions of others to help him adapt to everyday experiences. Understanding the child's spectrum of living at home, in school and in the community will point the way towards correcting social inadequacies and imbalances. Processes of social influence involving interests, gestures, skills and other behavior are learned and maintained through imitation and intuition and continued throughout adolescence. Youth plays two social roles, child to his parents and friend to his peers; the presumed resolution of conflicts in favor of the latter is exaggerated for there is little if any independence pain in parental cleavage.

The adolescent social development is determined by the social setting and socioeconomic status. Farm adolescents differ from town adolescents and from urban adolescents according to the opportunities available for social experiences and time utilization. Cultural modes of behavior which increase the opportunity for boys and girls to socialize diminish emotional tension, whereas restricted association with the opposite sex increases emotional stress. But some parents increase pressure drives on adolescents to experience drives to a greater degree than cultural customs permit. The adolescent is caught between wanting his needs fulfilled and wanting to be accepted as a grown-up, adequate to fulfill his own needs. At one time, he is ready to accept the same responsibility from his parents as in the past, but at another time wants to throw off his home dependence. He shows similar vascillation in his play with peers, swinging from active energetic play to inactive sophisticated interests, ever confusing to parents.

The major adolescent problem is his relationship to the opposite sex and to love objects; his first interest is love of self and those like him. He has strong friendships but always remains self-centered; he is not interested in helping others but appears considerate of everyone in his orbit. Yet, building up a self-image of a satisfactory adult becomes the prime objective of his social development. From the love of self and of others like himself he gradually turns to love of a person outside the family, usually one of the same sex. Between thirteen and fifteen, he worships heroes; the girl has crushes on an older woman. It is a safe experience because it directs his interest towards individuals outside the family and to persons far removed from himself. It is a transference feeling from the parent to another adult idol to which he relates with strong feelings of affection, an experience that leads to the development of love relationships. From the love of hero worship, most adolescents gradually turn to the opposite sex with overt shyness and subtle antagonism. Some become withdrawn and moody and want to be left alone to relax from the social strains of adolescence. Heterosexual interests in older persons of the opposite sex begin at fifteen, despite rebuffs from the family, until gradual interest in members of the opposite sex of the same age evolves, with one relationship at a time. Both boys and girls are still shy and awkward, glance at each other obliquely, stray off into corners to hold hands, share confidences, plan their lives together and become dependent socially on each other. It marks the beginning of kissing and petting and the kind of personal games that bring the sexes together. In mid-adolescence boys begin to wisecrack to gain attention in order to cover up self-consciousness; others remain blasé; and still others talk about things beyond their knowledge. Romantic relationships are short but intense and end suddenly with petty quarreling and rapid recovery. Some have many intense relationships in rapid sequence; others unprepared to relate to the opposite sex unconsciously keep themselves obese, unclean and unkempt; still others turn to physical complaints, real or imagined, as an excuse for not participating with their peers; and a few continue to carry on with members of the same sex cultivating homosexuality as a lifelong pattern. Many overemphasize their school work, seek the commendation of teachers and parents as a substitute for social success with the opposite sex, tendencies symptomatic of difficulties in heterosexual adjustment.

Adolescents identify with their own peer groups, imitate them in behavior and plan their goals together. But adolescents under stringent parental restrictions feel differently and resent the limitations. The wholesome peer group wants its members to be good sports, have a good sense of humor, to do well in school, appear attractive and be good dancers. The wayward peer group of hippies demands stoic acceptance of inflicted pain, gang warfare, sex practices, planned theft and other proofs of gang solidarity. Some groups interested in sports, ecology or extracurricular activities will absorb the adolescent's time in meaningful ways. However, membership in gangs may have destructive results on youngsters' efforts to socialize. Youth may develop interest in hold-ups, larceny, warfare that constitute juvenile delinquency. Many efforts are being made to work with these groups to meet their need for excitement through socially acceptable channels.

Social Adjustment

The adolescent years are characterized by social development and adjustment in a small clique of an equal number of active boys and girls. The activities of the group vary from one season to another, providing experience for getting along with other people, developing loyalty to the group, helping emancipation from home and culture, cultivating the art of lovemaking under protective circumstances, all with the feeling of peer approval and social belonging. Peer culture is the summum bonum of spontaneous social manifestations during mid-adolescence when peer values have greater effect than adult values. The social entente encourages snobbery, creating intense rivalry with outbreaks of violence between groups. Nevertheless, the group does more to bring about normal social growth than do parents and teachers combined. The clique, the fraternity and sorority are less healthy emotionally and socially than community peer groups. Adolescents go to extremes in social adulation and social ostracism amongst them but the group is intolerant of wealth or socioeconomic status, demands loyalty from its members, and blocks beneficial social contacts from without.

Social acceptance or rejection of an individual by a group is a complex phenomenon. Each youth selects from his schoolmates one or two whom he admires, prefers to work with, likes to play with, and chooses as an intimate friend and relies on him as a dependable companion. Appearance and manners determine social acceptance—an attractive face, a slim figure, a pleasing manner, fluent talk, stylish hairdo, approved clothes are admired traits. Homeliness, dirtiness, or thinness, excessive perspiration, hesitant speech, crude manners, out-of-date clothes are current sources of unpopularity. Adolescents are tremendously sensitive to social stimuli, for no other problem seems so important as establishing themselves in their own society. The traits admired by adolescents are established, hence it is possible to measure the social adjustment of the youth to determine which phases of his life are adequate and which inadequate in his adaptation to society.

Parents must learn to maintain a consistent attitude during the adolescent's progression in social development. Youth needs to feel that in his family there are firm standards and limits which continue in spite of occasional relaxation. Wholesome family standards of behavior will constitute positive guides to him throughout maturation. He needs to feel, too, that his parents will support him in spite of his failures in social and sexual adjustment. Living with adolescents is continuous excitement charged with new and different problems. An understanding of what youth is experiencing in social development will be stimulating to both parents and teachers. Clearly, the conflicts of adolescents should be seen as manifestations of organizing social development rather than absurd personal behavior.

Social normality is determined by the extent an individual

elicits social responses similar to those of most people. The total social responses may yield a net surplus, deficit or zero. The average human remains invisible and so youth is unkempt, unclean, unsavory to become visible. If we construct a continuum running from one extreme of social restrictions of the institutionalized to the opposite extreme of social abettment of the self-actualized, we find both groups socially visible. They behave in ways that always attract attention but in the middle of the continuum the behavior of most people hardly impels society to respond in any way. The average thus constitutes the normal individuals who conform to salient social expectations, revealing little about their distinguishing characteristics. Each of the three groups includes extroverted and introverted youths; the former condition poorly, and so require a good deal of firmness in their management, while the latter condition well and might be harmed by excessive severity. The attempts of society to treat both types alike probably mean straddling between two stools and getting the worst of both. Cursory qualitative judgments of social behavior will prevail until sociality is quantitated. Social age is a definite measure that will take its place with intellectual and emotional age as an index of maturation at any age.

Peer Status

The most significant personality change during adolescence is the diminished status an individual derives from the dependent relationship to parents with a corresponding increase in the primary status earned in his own right. The adolescent gains intrinsic self-esteem independent of his status in the peer group by achieving acceptance, by subordinating himself to group interests, by making himself dependent on group approval. The peer group relieves the loss of anchorage to the home in early adolescence by providing relief from uncertainty, indecision and anxiety about proper ways of thinking, feeling and behaving. The organized group excludes adults to liberate youth from their controls, rejects the accepted adult standards and becomes the major force in resisting acculturation in society. The peer group provides the media for heterosexual gratification and the norms of sex behavior, reduces frustrations and stabilizes the long transitional period, offers compensations for deprivations from ethnic, racial or religious affiliations. Little privations are easily endured when the heart and mind are better treated than the body.

Youth is shaped by the culture, by society and by the people around him. When he joins a group, his life is enriched and expanded, his strength increased, his courage extended, his objectives solidified, his personal worth established. He receives an income of friendliness, approval, recognition, and returns the compliments to others in the group—he gets and gives. But there are limitations; the individual cannot do what he pleases. The group defines his role indicating approval or disapproval, good or bad, loyal or disloyal and the status of the individual becomes crystallized. Conformity, recognition and success are the bywords of the group where everyone craves the anesthetizing security of being identified with the majority. Youth is half ruined by conformity and would be wholly ruined without it. Adolescents are created different; they lose their social freedom and their individual autonomy in seeking to become like each other.

Group membership may not be a developmental asset. The family circle sometimes has a destructive effect on an individual member when rejected, intimidated, or over-disciplined. Peer groups outside the home may have detrimental effects on some of their members. School groups under adult supervision may achieve good social growth. But spontaneous youth groups may be too authoritarian—reject a member who fails in group activities, ostracize one who differs in appearance, status, race and religion, intimidate one critical of group standards. No adolescent can have society upon his own terms; if he seeks it, he must serve it too. American social life constitutes an evasion of talking to people; most Americans don't really get together; they only do things together. But youth groups discourse, cooperate, compete and compromise together. Belongingness to the group replaces family ties, hence the adolescent's dependence on the esteem of his peers. Group memberships mediate the transition from the family member to the independent maturing adult. Group relations may cause social isolation when youth fails to receive the educative benefits of membership, for social enslavement makes youth respond so automatically to expectations that he develops no stable sense of self. These maladaptive consequences of group participation thus impede cultivation of a clear-cut self-image of adolescent personality.

Interacting with others in groups is a necessary educative experience but not a sufficient social stimulus. One of the attributes of maturity is to sustain intimate relations with very close friends. Public behavior in groups does not provide the private conditions essential for intimacy, confidence and aspirations. Close friendships are indispensable for the growth and integration of personality in understanding one's self and others and cultivating loving relationships. Puberal girls break away from dependence upon parents by developing a strong urge for secrecy with another girl for ego maturation rather than for exotic satisfaction. Identification with another girl strengthens the consciousness of her independent ego. Close friendships discover and define the self; group competitions crystallize into a clear sense of one's social competence; private experiences unravel personal worth, neutralizing fears about meeting group standards, airing hopes and aspirations for the future. Once the desire for intimacy shifts to a member of the opposite sex, youth gradually arrives at a concept of his identity by projecting his diffused ego images on another and beholds the crystallized reflections of the confused ego.

Adolescent friendships become charged with strong emotionality that helps correct faults in past social experiences. The friend takes on new meaning for the interests of one become equal to the other. It creates a wholesome approach to interrelationships, transferring the immature getting attitude of, "What shall I do to get what I want" to the mature giving attitude, "What shall I do to contribute to the feeling of worthwhileness of my friend." Such is the composition of love even without overt sexual activity for true mutuality. Not all friendships are wholesome. Sometimes one dominates the other, exploits the other, criticizes the other. Mismatched friendships produce wariness, withdrawal, weariness. The strong and the weak cannot keep company together. Nevertheless, socialization—private and public—must be encouraged to learn of people and their ways. In the confusion, youth develops many casual acquaintances, but no real friends to unravel the self in relation to others. Youth is known by the company he organizes.

Youth Subculture

Human life is reduced to suffering when two ages, two cultures overlap. The affluence of a wealthy society can maintain a large segment of its idle adolescent population of over 25 million without productivity. The subculture is identified by a distinctive style of dress, special vocabulary, leisure attitudes, unique periodicals, entertainment idols and weird music. Great value is placed on fun, leisure, attractiveness and popularity. The summum bonum of human life is happiness, for means and ends are measured by how much they contribute to or detract from happiness. Happiness is what we have divided by what we think we ought to have. The peer groups have little for both numerator and denominator and so they remain happy for the moment. Group conformity rejects adult authority and suppressed individuality in a clique atmosphere characterized by restlessness, boredom and excitement. The youth subculture is a by-product of the tasks confronting the maturing adolescent abounding in great reservoirs of physical and mental energy that demand action, excitement and experimentation, in new sexual drives that bewilder him and unsettle his sense of identity. He is in an unstable state not yet emancipated from the dependency of childhood, craving for direction, assurance and approval. He is not fully cognizant of the future, trying to establish some link with the world, some means of identity with larger activities, and some challenge beyond the boundaries of self.

All adolescent impulses and needs, whether forbidden or disintegrative, cannot be openly expressed else they will lead to an inevitable clash with society. Yet all impulses and needs that are mastered and controlled, but not expressed, will not lead to a clash with social values. On the other hand, forbidden disintegrative needs and impulses converted into accepted actions and openly expressed may also lead to a clash with society. But this kind of conflict with the establishment constitutes constructive maturation. If the integrated youth is directed from his inner resources to clash with external values, this is his decision; he is not driven to it.

Adult society accounts for some of youth's subculture. Experience and understanding are their rather abstract god-figures and ignorance and stupidity make them angry. Our universities are their religious training centers; our libraries, museums, art galleries, theatres, concert halls and sports arenas are their place of communal worship. Commercial interests foster excessive spending and unique buying habits via their own youth publications and communication media. There is a void in modern society to serve the role of youth, in marked contrast to agrarian society where youth plays an active role in the family economy. Other deleterious forces foster this subculture: materialism, abandonment of religious and puritanical ethics, displacement of work and saving by leisure and spending.

Freudian ethics of permissiveness and sexuality is another social force for realizing an integrated personality. Finally, there is adult abdication from guiding the young with respect to a positive approach to life and a negative degradation of drug addiction, cigarette smoking, sexual promiscuity, and other disintegrating vices of man. Adolescent subculture will lead to social decay if youth is not guided towards personal destiny. He must learn to combine freedom with respect for others, with personal regard for the consequences of his actions. He must be subject to rigorous intellectual discipline, ever challenged in all his vital activities. He must have adult love and support throughout the maturing years, learn to derive satisfaction from intangibles such as accomplishment, integrity, service, and self-respect, justice, charity, with reverence for human life.

Adolescent Alienation

Biological adolescence begins several years earlier than a century ago because of improved nutrition and health, but social adolescence is delayed for years with increasing technological development of industrial society. The mastery of adult roles during this new postadolescence requires a prolonged prelude that allows adolescent affairs which ripen some and rot others. The lame in the path outstrip the swift who wander from it; chance favors only those who know how to court her. Youth completed the psychological preparation for maturity with emancipation from parents, comfort with sexuality, attainment of identity and capacity for intimacy, but mandatory schooling shelters him from work responsibility in society. It is different from the Middle Ages when the child of seven was assimilated into the adult world by apprenticeship without formal education. He was led into the family work path by severity, not by persuasion as we do today, using soft words as hard arguments. But youth is better persuaded by the reasons which they have themselves discovered than by those which have come into the minds of their elders. It robs so much flowering time for youth to do something and be somebody.

Adolescent confusion is the current designation for apparent order which is not understood. The questions posed by youth show the mind's range and answers its subtlety. There is so much more to be learned from the unexpected questions than from the discourses of elders, who talk in rote according to notions they borrowed and prejudices they acquired from training and education. The great pleasure of ignorance is the pleasure of asking questions. The adult who has lost this pleasure or exchanged it for the pleasure of dogma, the pleasure of answering, is already beginning to stiffen. Youth is questioning the very foundation of society before enrolling as participants. That stirs the very inners in many, producing moods of euphoria hopeful of instituting harmony, beauty and idealism in a discordant world while stirring moods of alienation in others in despair of any hope for an ugly world. Youth declares that they will not enter into society to become worse than they were before, nor to have fewer rights than they had before, but to have these rights better secured. They will not become bound to a society which robs them of a part of their very essence and replaces it with a speck of the gigantic personality which is its own. They see only what they know. Their vision is limited and their knowledge meager. They lack the knack of transforming vague ambition into effective tactics. But they must plan their own strategy with indirect help of one in the chosen field; they must work with some clear objective for a life career in view and remain alert to seize unexpected opportunities.

Contemporary youth is greatly concerned with the irrational phases of the adult world in order to change society, control objectives and correct corruption. On the surface the dissent appears sound but it may represent an externalization from inner irrational forces, an unrealistic or unproductive approach, a formulation of problems without solutions. It is basically a normal developmental phenomenon in achieving physical and psychologic distance from parents and society via many movements. When all are alienated together they're no longer lonely. Clinically, adolescents may be individually or collectively disturbed, expressed in alienation, the state of our society and culture. In intellectualization, the body and its needs are almost totally disregarded to exalt the intellect to its proper place. Intellectualization is regarded as the characteristic defense of the adolescent until activity comes to the fore to act out in groups for changes sought in society. Youth rejects all ideologies, capitalist and communist alike. They insist on unconditional morality now, an immediate change with total disdain for tactics and practicality, on substitution of rhetoric for hard work, irresponsible calls for social revolution that endanger the very possibility of change.

The pathological syndrome of alienation is manifested by living in the present without commitment to people, causes or ideas; by lack of communication with parents and other adults; by failure to concentrate on school or work tasks; by confused sense of identity and/or self-concept; by promiscuous ungratified sexual behavior; by drug addiction to marijuana or heroin; by sudden attacks of depression accompanied by attempts at suicide. The syndrome may be precipitated internally by rebellion against authority, by fear of success or failure, by a feeling of being unloved, and externally by the rapid rates of social change and human values, by perpetration of boring automation, by the isolation of generations. To live is to feel one's self lost; he who accepts it has already begun to find himself, to be on firm ground.

REFERENCES

Adelman, J. *et al.*: Growth of political ideas in adolescence. *J. Pers. Soc. Psychol.*, *4*:295-306, 1966.

Allee, W. C.: *Cooperation Among Animals.* New York, Abelard, 1951.

Aring, C. D.: In respect of youth. *Arch. Intern. Med.*, Vol. 124, 1969.

Astin, A. W. *et al.*: Life goals and vocational choice. *J. Appl. Psychol.*, *48*: 50-58, 1964.

Bandura, A. *et al.*: *Social Learning and Personality Development.* New York, Holt, Rinehart & Winston, 1967.

Barbero, C. J. *et al.*: Environmental failure to thrive. *J. Pediatr.*, *71*:639, 1967.

Berman, G. *et al.*: Psychosocial aspects of academic achievement. *Am. J. Orthopsychiatry*, *41*:406-15, 1971.

Braceland, F. J.: The twentieth century adolescent. *Am. J. Psychoanal.*, *31*: 3-13, 1971.

Brenner, J. H. *et al.*: *Drugs and Youth.* New York, Liveright, 1970.

Buss, A. H.: *The Psychology of Aggression.* New York, Wiley, 1961.

Butterfield, E. C. *et al.*: The effects of differing institutional climates on the effectiveness of social reinforcement in the mentally retarded. *Am. J. Ment. Defic.*, *70*:48, 1965.

Cameron, D. C.: Youth and drugs. *J.A.M.A.*, *206*:1267-71, 1968.

Campbell, R.: Violence in adolescence. *J. Anal. Psychol.*, *12*:161-73, 1967.

Clausen, J. A. *et al.*: *Socialization and Society.* Boston, Little, Brown, 1968.

Coleman, J. S. *et al.*: *The Adolescent Society.* Glencoe, Free Press, 1961.

Coon, C.: Young people and society. *Practitioner*, *206*:275-7, 1971.

Doll, E. A.: *Vineland Social Maturity Scale.* Minneapolis, Educational Test Bureau, 1946.

Edgerton, R.: *The Cloak of Competence.* Berkeley, University California Press, 1967.

Eisner, V.: Alienation of youth. *J. Sch. Health*, *39*:81-90, 1969.

Erikson, E.: *Childhood and Society.* New York, Norton, 1968.

Frank, H. M. *et al.*: *Your Adolescent at Home and in School.* New York, Viking, 1956.

Glaser, K.: Conflicts and rebellion during adolescence. *Pediatrics*, 1960.

Glueck, S. & E.: *Unraveling Juvenile Delinquency.* New York, Commonwealth Fund, 1950.

Glueck, S. *et al.*: *Ventures in Criminology.* Cambridge, Harvard, 1964.

Goldstein, H.: Social and occupational adjustment. In H. A. Stevens and R. Heber (Eds.): *Mental Retardation.* Chicago, University Chicago Press, 1964.

Gunn, A. D. G.: *The Privileged Adolescent.* Medical and Technical Publishing, 1970.

Hess, R. D. *et al.:* The status of adolescents in American society. A problem of social identity. *Child Dev., 28:*459-468, 1957.

Kalimo, E.: *Determinants of Medical Care Utilization.* Helsinki, Institute Social Security, 1969.

Kappelman, M. M.: The adolescent and his dangers. *Clin. Pediatr., 10:*154-9, 1971.

Katz, J.: Adolescence and antisocial behavior. *Med. J. Aust., 1:*256-8, 1967.

Livingston, H. D.: Problems of adolescent development and social adaptation. *N. Z. Med. J., 64:*18, 1965.

Maddox, G. *et al.:* Overweight as social deviance and disability. *J. Health Soc. Behav., 9:*287-298, 1968.

Masterson, J. F. Jr.: The psychiatric significance of adolescent turmoil. *Am. J. Psychiatr., 124:*1549-54, 1968.

Matkom, A. J.: Impression formation as a function of adjustment. *Psychol. Monogr., 77:*1-19, 1963.

McKay, H. D.: Social influence on adolescent behavior. *J.A.M.A.,* p. 643, Nov. 1962.

Mechanic, D.: *Medical Sociology.* Glencoe, Free Press, 1968.

Miller, E.: Individual and social approach to the study of adolescence. *Br. J. Md. Psychol., 35:*211, 1962.

Murphy, L. B.: *The Widening World of Childhood.* New York, Basic Books, 1962.

Offer, D.: Rebellion and antisocial behavior. *Am. J. Psychoanal., 31:*13-9, 1971.

Peterson, D. R.: *The Clinical Study of Social Behavior.* New York, Appleton-Century-Crofts, 1968.

Pfeiffer, E.: *Disordered Behavior.* New York, Oxford University Press, 1968.

Philips, I. *et al.:* Conformity, rebellion and learning: confrontation of youth with society. *Am. J. Orthopsychiatry, 40:*3, 1970.

Pond, D. A.: Behavior disorders of the adolescent. *Trans. Med. Soc. London, 86:*116-21, 1970.

Rezler, A. G.: The joint use of the Kuder preference record and the Holland VPI in the vocational assessment of high school girls. *Psychol. Sch., 4:* 81-84, 1967.

Rigg, C. A.: On communicating with teenagers. *Aust. Paediatr. J., 6:*17, 1970.

Robins, L.: *Deviant Children Grown Up.* Baltimore, Williams & Wilkins, 1966.

Rothney, J. W. M. *et al.: Guidance of American Youth.* Cambridge, Harvard University Press, 1950.

Ryle, A.: Problems in understanding adolescents. *Proc. Roy. Soc. Med., 71:* 512-4, 1968.

Schachter, S.: *The Psychology of Affiliation.* Stanford, Stanford University Press, 1959.

Schechter, M. D. *et al.:* Violence in adolescence. *Postgrad. Med., 45:*190-5, 1969.

Shapiro, D.: *Neurotic Styles.* New York, Basic Books, 1965.

Smith, E. A.: *American Youth Culture. Group Life in Teenage Society.* New York, Free Press, 1962.

Stott, D. H.: *Studies of Troublesome Children.* London, Tavistock, 1966.

Tennent, T. G.: Truancy and stealing. *Br. J. Psychiatry, 116:*587-92, 1970.

Thomas, A. *et al.: Temperament and Behavior Disorders in Children.* New York, New York University Press, 1968.

Tuma, E. *et al.:* Family socioeconomic status and adolescent attitudes to authority. *Child Dev., 31:*387-399, 1960.

Ullmann, L. P. *et al.: Case Studies in Behavior Modification.* New York, Holt, Rinehart & Winston, 1965.

Vail, D.: *Dehumanization and the Institutional Career.* Springfield, Thomas, 1966.

Weigert, E.: Basic factors of human existence. *Psychiatry, 23:*121-131, 1960.

Wesselius, L. F.: Behavior problems in adolescents. *J. Med. Soc. N. J., 65:*498-503, 1968.

Winnicott, F. R. C. P.: Adolescent process and the need for personal confrontation. *Pediatrics, 44:*752, 1969.

Wise, L. J.: Alienation of present-day adolescents. *J. Am. Acad. Child Psychiatry, 9(2):*264-277, 1970.

Yates, A. J.: *Behavior Therapy.* New York, Wiley, 1970.

CHAPTER VI

SEXUAL IMMATURITY

Each loves itself, but not itself alone,
Each sex desires alike, 'til two are one,
Nor ends the pleasure with the fierce embrace;
They love themselves a third time in the race.

Sex is the core of human power, the medium for expressing emotional impulses, the mover of all we do and dream. There is the sensual sexuality that culminates in orgasm via coitus, masturbation or perversion. There is the mature, genuine, unselfish love—the gift of one's self, the true flow of life—whose roots are deep in the earth and whose branches extend into heaven. There is the instinct to mate that meets reason half-way to have the long, steady, reliable companionship that brings comfort and encouragement in whatever happens, and loyalty, as true as a dial to the sun, of the one of choice of the opposite sex. Then there is all of the deep-seated devotion, moral responsibility and fruitful endeavor to troublesome children in a sacred family of one's creation. Sex potential acquired at puberty in an immature physical, emotional and social organism is completely out of its mileu for it takes adequate and balanced maturity of body and mind and spirit to articulate this great gift of life to the fullest benefit of both partners.

Sexuality is built into the brain, not just shaped by emotional experience and sustained by the trickle of hormones from the sexual glands. Male and female brains are different, but manhood has to assert itself in the normal development of the male brain and if nothing intervenes in the form of male hormone, the brain will be female. The single individual is only half a person for normal life is shaped by interactions with a mate and the more interpersonal, the more effective the total homeostasis of the sex bond. It is the man and woman united that make the complete human being. The sex drive is organized in the central sites of the brain while love and other emotions are generated in the larger regions. The sex emotion in concert with all others

189

is a powerful instrument of social life manifested by charm and charisma. The phenomenon that men and women are born with markedly different emotional tendencies makes women, man's confusion.

Lack of Sexual Standards

Ancient eros is coming into its own. This is the age of liberalism; it involves the use of the body at the behest of the head. The essence of the liberal outlook lies not in what opinions are held, but in how they are held; instead of being held dogmatically, they are held tentatively, with the consciousness that new evidence may lead to their abandonment. That enables us to put aside our culturally acquired principles for objective outlooks on normal and deviant sexual behavior. Current concepts must be correlated with the value system of contemporary society, for the heterodoxy of one age is the orthodoxy of the next. Sexual behavior is so intimately entwined with moral issues, religious sentiments and cultural concepts that any liberal approach is deemed immoral or illegal. Such narrow-souled folks are like narrow-necked bottles; the less they have in them, the more noise they make in pouring it out. The settled point of view is the more fatal illusion; since life is growth and motion, a fixed point of view kills anybody who has one. If you look at life in one way, there is always cause for alarm.

Attitudes about morality, virginity, fidelity, love, marriage and sexual behavior are meaningful only within the context of the cultural and religious mores. In the first century of the Christian Era nudity was no cause for shame, virginity was not prized, fidelity nonexistent, marriage temporary. Open sexuality was the rule, incest was frequent, women invited intercourse. Even at the wedding ceremony the guests would copulate with the bride. Sexual freedom was gradually curtailed by church regulation of sex behavior as the greatest solution for public ills. The more the church enforced sexual taboos by cruel exactions, the more sexual perversions ensued and guilt about sexuality became universal. Christianity gave Eros poison to drink; he did not die of it, but degenerated into vice. Somehow, the sexually free societies remained relatively free from sexual perversion. Even the homosexuals of the early Greeks exercised the pattern of bisexuality in which homosexual feelings were considered as natural as heterosexual ones. It was not until the twelfth century that the ideal of love and love for marriage evolved in Western civilization as an institution founded upon an instinct for the mingling of love, friendship, sensuality and respect. Civilized people cannot fully satisfy their sexual instinct without love.

The sexual act goes far beyond the reproductive function. It is not just an exchange of nuclear material between cells of mating types or sexes. Reproduction has validity for primitive forms of life but not for the human being who evolves with multiple sex-related activities. Man's inherent psychosexual neutrality at birth permits the development of varied psychosexual functions that lead to diverse sexual behavior. Arousal and response are determined by situational and learning factors to such an extent that the individual may seek gratification in homosexual objects if no human being is available. Even the physiological root of gratification through the genital or other erotogenic zone is conditioned by experience affected by age, health, fatigue, nutrition and recency of drive fulfillment. Sexuality is self-limiting if it is satisfactory; it diminishes tension and clears the mind for attention in learning far better than sex abstainers who run away from what they desire but carry their desires with them.

The bisexual anlage of the human embryo leads to the bisexual tendency at a psychological level. It is observed in latent homosexual manifestations in affectionate feelings for members of one's own sex and in behavior patterns characteristics of the opposite sex, i.e. artistic or culinary interests in males or athletic or scientific interests in females. The final shaping of the normal individual, however, reveals no double embryonic origin of the genital system reflected in sexual duality. Biological sex is clearly differentiated at the moment of conception by the XX and XY chromosomal patterns, but the presence of androgens and estrogens in both male and female blood serves only for growth and maturity of the primary genital system and for the development of secondary sexual characteristics without affecting sexuality. And the strength of the sexual impulse in a man does not depend upon the proportion of masculinity in his composition any more than the degree of feminity in a woman determines her sexual impulse. These differences are subject to growth, development and maturation with a mate of choice in sexual harmony. The sexual instinct is always active in woman but at rest from time to time in man.

There is clearly no primary genetic mechanism to preordain masculinity or feminity of psychosexual differentiation. The patterning of sexual behavior begins at birth with many cues stimulating gender role expectations until the core gender identity is established at age three and reinforced throughout childhood by certain human traits socially specialized as the appropriate attitudes and behavior of each sex. This social specialization becomes rationalized into the clinical theory that the socially decreed behavior is natural for one sex and unnatural for the other, and that the deviant develops as a result of a congenital, endocrine or developmental disorder. Deviance from the group norms of "increase and multiply" was threatening to the continuity of early society with marginal survival. It is no longer so with the population explosion approaching doomesday by A.D. 3000. The range of permissible deviance in sex is thus related to individual life styles limited to decadent elites. The oral contraceptive produced changes in conceptual attitudes and value systems of modern society. Sexual perversions are giving way to sexual deviation and to sexual variation. The wide spectrum of patterns in sexual behavior in the privacy of the bedroom thus violates rigid conventional standards. Certainly nothing is unnatural that is not physically impossible and everything goes in the intimacy of sex relations.

The habitual deviant has difficulty in achieving satisfactory sexual relations with a mature partner of the opposite sex as a result of disturbed family relations, impaired gender-identity development, poor ego cultivation, unconscious fear, hate or guilt. Healthy sexuality with a discriminating partner seeks erotic satisfaction in the context of affection by giving and receiving pleasure. Pathologic sexuality with a nondiscriminating partner seeks relief from nonsexual tension by excessive neurotic giving and taking.

Every human being becomes transparent in the life style of his sexual relationships in his pattern of personality. The style of life formed in childhood adapts to three great forces in adolescence—sex, occupation, society, the SOS of each individual. If youth is hampered by structural or functional inferiority in making any of these adaptations there are three possibilities: success, neurosis or disease. For body as for soul, there is the effort that overcomes weakness and leads to strength, the hesitation and compromise that means evasion of difficulty and leads to neurosis, and the despairing retreat that entails frank disaster.

Lack of Sexual Capacity

Sexual inadequacy, real or virtual, is the bane of adolescent life. How shall one who is so weak in childhood become really strong in adolescence? He only changes his fancies about satisfactory feelings and attitudes toward sex. Some boys doubt their masculinity, prove it to themselves by aberrant behavior; some girls find the prospect of becoming a woman frightening and persist in tomboyish behavior. They need to know more about the issues, values and interpersonal relationships rather than reproductive facts. There must be a weakening of innate fear to evoke real understanding of deterrents, of cultural intermingling, of changing sex roles, of scientific inquiry, of conflicting standards. The determining factor in sexual behavior is neither the tremendous power of the sex drive nor the intellectual decision; for the adolescent who feels that he is progressing in life objectives has no difficulty in managing his sexual impulses in a socially approved way. But the promiscuous youth, the individual who is using sex exploitively is seeking satisfactions through sex which he could not find in other more acceptable ways. These adolescents usually emerge from backgrounds charged with conflict, rejection and failure. They remain incompetent, inadequate and incongruous in sex relations, denying themselves their birthright to a full life while inviting cryptogenic and/or psychosomatic ailments, self-induced from postmasturbation conflicts and/or experimental heterosexual frustrations.

Sex is a composite of at least seven of these fundamental determinants—nuclear, pituitary, sex glands, hormonal status, external genitalia, internal genitalia, birth sex and total upbringing. The latter is usually decisive despite any discrepancy in all other variables. The love life of man must permeate the whole personality so that all levels of expression participate in its full realization. The whole being must lose himself completely in the experience, a goal only possible through optimal maturation. The sexual function of an adolescent cannot be considered as an isolated entity. It is a part of the whole which must function in its entirety or not at all. If youth endows some phases of sex activity with awe and guilt, all the components of the background of that activity will be similarly clothed. Anything happening to an adolescent in one sphere of his activity will have its reverberations in all spheres. Mental and emotional disorders emerging in conflict over sexual matters will be expressed in body language, although emotional problems related to sex difficulties may assume many disguises.

Adjusted youth seeks love because it brings ecstasy; it relieves loneliness; and in the union of love it reveals in a mystic miniature, the prefiguring vision of the heaven that saints and poets have long imagined. Then, too, the adolescent finds a way of expressing manly emotions through sex—dependency, sadism, masochism, nurture and rebellion, and love, affection, tenderness and occasionally transcendency and mystical union with the universe. Sex will sometimes express one combination of drives and sometimes another, hence each act is unique in the way the union is consummated. It is not a matter of physical technique but a matter of psychic expression of one for another. Any analysis of the act into its components inhibits spontaneous expression of emotions bound in it, but theoretically it is subject to analysis.

The sex act is not only a physical union of two beings but a bio-physicochemical-emotional reaction between two different systems integrating their all for the very personal encounter. Such integration is usually difficult because the two beings bring to the act their own heterogeneous accretions of infantile attachments, childish conditioning, parental indoctrination, moral structure, religious injunctions, social taboos and polyglot love patterns that thwart the intensity, duration and totality of the reaction from inhibitory overtones. After all, sex energy is more powerful than nuclear energy. And the more these extraneous forces within each being are suppressed during the prelude, the more effective the exothermic reaction that subdues the two participants to unique relaxation with a sublime feeling of human transcendence. It contrasts so markedly with the end feeling that befalls immature humans given to rooster release and its concomitant sexual deviations.

Adolescent immaturity is expressed in sexual as well as in all other aspects of everyday life by the inability to make mature decisions during a lifetime of endless childhood devoid of identity. Falling in love gives them adult images but that love is usually the distorted concept created by commercial communication. The male reaches his greatest physical sexual potential between sixteen and eighteen years with a variable plateau for life while the female sex drive is not truly manifest until the early twenties, despite pretenses, and persists longer than in the male. Sexual symbiasis depends on sexual communication. Each partner must understand the demands and/or desires of the other to avoid a break in the bond or development of psychosomatic disorder. Most problems in the sexual area are manifestations of a breakdown in communication, loss of respect and responsibility, guilt feelings based on taboos. Failure may be due to communication with their image of the partner rather than the partner's image of self. If such communication insults rather than fortifies the ego, it is due to the difference in individual concepts of themselves and each other—real or imagined.

Lack of Functional Effectiveness

Sexual disturbances in adolescents may be due to relative ignorance of one or both partners, poor fit between them, or psychopathology in one or both participants. Every sexual problem usually embodies all these factors. Common adolescent complaints involve inadequate sexual drive, ineffective sexual responsivity, abnormal sex practices, persistent masturbation, coital discord, psychosomatic disorder. The perception of the problem is far more significant than the reality. All aspects of the individual sex life must be unravelled, interpreted and corrected to assuage body and mind. After all, the sex instinct and its mode of gratification are prime movers of all youth does and dreams. Developmental failure of the sex impulse produces a variety of anomalous sexual behavior.

Masturbation guilt in young adolescents creates internal turmoil that threatens equilibrium. The sexual drive creates fantasy about the means of satisfaction, hence the development of healthy or unhealthy attitudes towards sex is largely controlled by prevailing psychological influences. The amount of physical masturbation at any given time is no index of the degree of mental health. We are a long way from the mistaken view that masturbation must not take place because it is very wrong; we know that it is a normal activity which attains its peak in adolescence. In fact, masturbation contributes to normal psychological development by giving youth the opportunity to experience sexual feelings within the temporary safety of his fantasies and thoughts. Some disturbed adolescents, however, experience extreme guilt and shame, and feel that they are harming their body and brain. Reassurance can help if their problem is made easy to discuss, otherwise formal psychotherapeutic help may be necessary.

Masturbation is more frequent in boys than in girls partly because of the male external genitalia and partly because boys are less stringent about doctrination in social circles. But this predominance of male masturbation over female masturbation is reversed in maturity because women have more exacting requirements for an orgasm than men. Lack of sufficient orgasm during intercourse and the psychological stimulus of incomplete coitus produce a masturbating or frigid woman, even though not all frigid women masturbate. Young women tend to have cycles of increased or decreased sexual urges which correlate with some phase of the menstrual cycle. Sexual desire is usually at its peak during the intermenstrual or ovulatory period, hence those with perfectly regular menses have regularly recurring cycles of maximal and waning sexual interest. There may also be regular alternations of increased and decreased sexual appetite with or without assumed cyclic alterations in young men. Highly sexed men and women create marked external expressions of intense sexual drives but physical expressions of sexual interests are not necessarily a direct function of the real strength of the sexual drive. The physiological state of the adolescent at any particular time is one of the most potent modifying factors of his basic sexual drive.

Sex-superiority complex in a muscular male subdues rather than stimulates his partner. He becomes a veritable rooster in the sex act with little foreplay, stretches the uterosacral ligaments by painful penetration in a poorly lubricated vagina, achieves his climax and gives the partner a backache. The pompous male is under the misconception that intensity of loving is a direct function of the size of the penis, that the female is available as a beneficent service, that full penetration affords him optimal satisfaction. He has no understanding of the differences in time required for male and female sexual responses, respectively. He pays little credence to it as a self-centered, immature egoist with minimal sexual capacity. In fact, he may continue in the same vein, exacting intercourse several times a day and causing vaginitis, vaginisms and frigidity. Egoism is the anesthetic that dulls the pain of stupidity. Marriage may qualify the fury of his passion but it rarely mends his manners—personal or pubic.

Premature ejaculation is due to failure to control the ejaculatory process long enough for intravaginal contact to satisfy the partner in half of his coital experiences. The woman's sexual intensity is increased by precoital sex play edged by the stimulation of penetration and so instantaneous ejaculation is frustrating, if repeated time after time. Such a functional pattern emerges from impromptu copulation with rapid intramission and quick ejaculation, from prolonged petting without any attempt to vaginalize penetration, or any thought given to the sexual tensions that ensue with such release, from quick withdrawal during the peak of the coital act without intravaginal ejaculation. The end result is that most young men never gain sufficient ejaculatory control to satisfy their partner. Premature ejaculation is excluded from the spectrum of impotence. It is not a part of the mechanism of conceptive and erective inadequacy for the premature ejaculator functions with a high degree of reproductive efficiency and unfortunately for the female partner, with little waste of time. Sexual dysfunction may be preceded by a prior state of premature ejaculation; acute ingestion of alcohol; maternal dominance that deprecates the young male's security in masculinity, with his father relegated to a second class citizen in the family structure. On the other hand, there may be cryptogenic impotence following paternal domineering with total obliteration of the female figure in the home; by religious orthodoxy with sexual function depersonalized for biologic reproduction; by homosexuality eliminating heterosexual dating.

Impotence or sex powerlessness frustrates; and absolute powerlessness frustrates absolutely. It is a dangerous emotion to initiate an independent life that needs adequate sex in that great amateur art to achieve optimal maturation. Impotence is a complicated problem that may be relative or complete and may involve any phase of the sexual act; there may be lack of interest in intercourse, inability to have or maintain an erection, premature or retarded ejaculation, or intercourse and ejaculation without orgasm. An adolescent male unable to maintain or achieve an erection necessary and sufficient for coital connection in either homosexual or heterosexual relationships requires physical and psychological probing. There is rarely complete lack of sexual response despite failure to develop an erection or attain an orgasm. Relative impotence occurs only under conditions of intercourse and does not interfere with morning erections, nocturnal emissions, or masturbation; absolute impotence may be due to emotional disturbance, endocrine dysfunction or neurologic lesion. The adolescent who complains of impotence or lack of libido may suffer from some hormonal lack while the eunuch with both impotence and absent libido complains of being mistaken for a girl over the phone.

Ineffective sexual functioning may be due to inborn constitutional factors influencing normal sexual development but parental oversolicitude, prohibitions, threats of castration are even more likely to inhibit the onset of the natural instinctive urge. Sex becomes taboo, a sense of shame and guilt is generated, and a mature heterosexual level blocked. Adolescent impotence may be based on regression or fixation for childhood experiences and reactions may have led to fear of masculine sexuality and its accompanying dangers and thus veer youth into the protective custody of an infantile state instead of the independence of a man. Or, the impotence may be due to fixation at a level before the development of strong masculine impulses that represent maturity, responsibility and sexuality, at variance with the lifelong orientation toward passivity. The sexual current is thus greatly influenced in both strength and quality by childish dependent trends.

Psychosocial restrictions may originate in religious orthodoxy, homosexual relations and prostitute devaluation. Religious teachings may indoctrinate the adolescent with the concept that overt sexual activity is sinful prior to marriage. Homosexual activity may contribute to coital failure in heterosexual relations. Drugs may alter the biophysical status for coital competence. Adolescent petting may evolve into disastrous trauma to the male ego aggravated by the girl's blind insistence that he do something. Traumatic episodes associated with the initial coital experience may establish a life style of sexual dysfunction. Nevertheless, many survive the stress of their initial opportunity for heterosexual coition, whether or not successful, and move into a continuity of effective sexual functioning in adulthood.

The woman considers orgasm a determining criterion of satisfaction in the coital act and craves for each coital experience simultaneously with the partner. Sexual satisfaction can be achieved by extended foreplay without pressure on either partner to proceed to coitus, by mutual mapping out of each partner's erogenic zone during protracted caressing sessions; by a more rostral male or a superior female position; by oral and manual stimulation of the penis or the clitoris as an integral part of coitus; by firm pressure on the dorsal and ventral aspects of the coronal sulcus just before ejaculation. Denial of sexual relationships as punishment for misdeeds and refusal to acknowledge pleasure from the sexual act are common ways of expressing rivalries—undercurrents for impotence and frigidity.

Frigidity is a misconcept of the female organic response, a man's accusation of a feeble reaction to his sexual feat. Once anxiety is suppressed and relaxation established there may be an occasional tumultuous release. The ingredients of a satisfying relationship are variety, spontaneity and consideration of each other's emotional desires. The inability to respond sexually at the conscious or subconscious levels is more virtual than real. Given the right partner and circumstances, any woman can achieve a satisfactory physical and emotional response. An emotional block is readily amenable to individual treatment for reinstating meaningful relationships by eliminating obstructive factors and feelings. A negative attitude toward the partner, anxiety about physical damage, a matrix of unwholesome attitudes from childhood, from parental warnings and from current folklore suppress sexual responsiveness. Rarely does orgasm failure follow stimulation of the clitoris and other vaginal erectile structures.

SEXUAL DEVIATIONS

Sexual deviations abound in the inadequate, immature youth because the community dictates sexual behavior and regulates mores, prohibitions and punishments. Certain sex practices are deemed sick and require medical correction even though the causes are no better understood today than they were a century ago. The intensity and direction of an adolescent's sexual desires and expressions cannot be labelled normal or abnormal but must be placed on a continuum. Very few individuals are always potent, invariably homosexual, or exclusively masochistic. There is probably no one who can have a satisfactory sexual relationship with any person in any manner at any time. Some are unwilling or unable to have a sexual relationship with any one at any time regardless of the manner; others restrict their behavior and their fantasy to one sex or style, and many of course to a single partner. Given a particular partner or situation, an individual is usually able to perform satisfactorily and with enjoyment; another may do so only rarely; and still another not at all.

Sexual behavior is influenced by mood, feeling, circumstance; sex ability, by desire, health, intensity, light or dark, naked or clothed, danger of discovery, and the biological cycle of the partner. Everyone has sexual interests that go beyond verto-ventral heterosexual coitus acceptable by society, but moral training, fear of consequences, availability of a willing partner and knowledge of techniques determine whether these desires are fulfilled.

Perverse Patterns

Sex deviates abound in an underprivileged or disturbed home unfilling basic adolescent needs and in an uncensored group lacking the moral standards of wholesome youth. Perverts, pimps and prostitutes are psychopathic individuals emanating from broken homes, possessive parents, unwanted progeny. Youth subjected to tremendous stimuli seek immediate gratification of sex needs, hence release of sexual tension becomes more important than choice for gratification. Youth emanating from difficult homes do not have the ego readiness to cope with heterosexual requisites of puberty, ever charged with fears of the opposite sex, doubts about sexual adequacy and images of hostile parental models.

Sexual perversion is usually a manifestation of psychosexual immaturity rather than of sexual, anatomic or constitutional disorders and interferes with the equilibration of the instinctive phases of sex and the total personality. The perverse adolescent seeks deviant sexual outlets because of an inability to obtain satisfaction in the mature love of another person of the opposite sex. Repetitive compulsive behavior relieves intolerable tensions for the moment and must be sought anew to satisfy infantile drives. Psychosexual immaturity is determined by unfavorable parental influence, unfortunate sexual experiences, persistent aggressiveness and destructiveness bound up with the sex instinct. True sexual deviation with profound personality disturbance arises from unconscious forces difficult to resist, even by skilled dynamic psychotherapy, while perverse sexual behavior remains completely under the individual's control. Youth hears that dark spirit of recalcitrance, always pulling him in the direction contrary to that in which he is reasonably expected to go. Perversion dominates sexual life in exhibitionism, sadism, masochism and transsexualism, or combinations of them, rare in women and in psychotics.

Sadism enhances sexual pleasure by inflicting physical cruelty during love play, intercourse or fantasy. Masochism enhances sexual pleasure by the subjective experience of pain ranging from mild to severe flagellation. Sexual fetishism for certain materials, such as Mackintosh, leather and silk, to augment sexual excitement leads to secret purchase of feminine underclothes, shoes, and apparel for self-stimulation. The sight and smell of girls so dressed enhances their sexual value for the satisfaction of intercourse. Transvestitism arouses sexual pleasure from wearing silky materials coupled with the idea of physical contact. It is ominous if perversion becomes a preferred substitute for normal sexual activity instead of an accompaniment. The more it is confined to fantasy and the less to performance, the better the prognosis.

Exhibitionism by an adolescent exposes his genitals to the opposite sex outside the context of the sexual act without the motive of intercourse. Genital exhibition occurs in both sexes in childhood as part of normal exploratory behavior, and in women of primitive societies. Simple exhibitionism follows sexual or social trauma, disappointment of a loved one, or severe mental or physical illness. The phobic type occurs in the amoral individual prone to other perversions and/or character disorders. Preconditioning develops normally in childhood but undergoes gradual repression, yet more adolescents expose themselves as a result of the intensity of sexual feelings and pride themselves on self-control and high moral standards in other spheres. The exhibitionist is like an infant who can neither tolerate tension nor wait for his needs to be satisfied but must be satisfied immediately. He avoids thinking, passes directly into action, and develops heightened self-esteem or narcissism.

Socophilia is pleasure in looking that leads to voyeurism, if restricted to the genitals. Such instincts become predominant in the phallic stage when curiosity about sexual matters is intensified. Libido from both oral and phallic stages finds a common pathway for expression and later in repression, with shyness as the reaction formation against socophilia. The eye becomes an erotogenic zone at age four when curiosity is greatly aroused. Coprolalia is the desire to have the sexual partner use profane language during the sexual act. It is an unconscious wish to degrade the woman yet serves as sex stimulation to attain the peak. Troilism is the desire for the sex partner to be shared with another person for invigorating the sex act. Pedophilia is the male erotic love of children to arouse the sex life of his youth in the face of sex inferiority. Urolagnea is sexual excitement associated with urinating upon someone and coprophilia is gratification from defecation as homosexual components.

Homosexuality

Sexual propensity for members of one's own sex varies in different individuals and even in the same individual during adolescence. Every sensitive adolescent may become preoccupied with his latent homosexuality. It is not an all or none condition, for all gradations exist between exclusive lifelong 100 percent homosexuality without any conscious capacity for arousal by heterosexual stimuli and exclusive 100 percent heterosexuality without any conscious capacity for homosexual stimuli. One-third of adolescents have some overt homosexual experience, but only 1 percent of all males are exclusively homosexual and 4 percent with both homosexual and heterosexual impulses. The homosexual act per se does not necessarily imply that the individual is predominantly homosexual in makeup. Situational homosexuality may be stimulated at school, camp, army installation and job corps center. Boys or girls may develop strong physical attractions for one another respectively and even develop love situations with indications that they are destined to become confirmed homosexuals. But real panic ensues upon realizing their response to a person of their own sex. Actually, situational homosexuality is transient and rarely binding unto real homosexuality. Once the setting changes, the pseudohomosexual bond wanes. A homosexual component exists in everybody, hence over one-third of the total male population may experience overt homosexual acts to the point of orgasm.

A satisfactory theory of homosexual behavior awaits our understanding the CNS mechanism of sexual arousal and learning forces that set the triggering devices for these personal actions. Curiously enough, we know less about heterosexual arousal as the natural phenomenon. Homosexuality is a complex with multiple causations: inappropriate identification with the opposite-sex parent, fear of or hostility to either parent, reversal of masculine and feminine roles in parents; feelings of inadequacy in males unable to fulfill sexual expectation, rigidity in dichotomy of male and female social roles with failure to allow for individuals who cannot fit into either of these roles; and easier access to sexual gratification with members of one's own sex in adolescence giving rise to chronic habit patterns. Seduction by adults has little effect in inducing homosexuality but may help to establish the pattern in a predisposed individual.

The adolescent male finds it difficult to achieve a normal identity in the midst of the diminishing importance of the father role in the home. Youth's evaluation for what is masculine or feminine in behavior plays a significant part in the adoption of inverted gender roles. More often the homosexual pattern develops through failure of heterosexual activity. A youth may have hatred of girls when disfiguring acne, obesity, dwarfism, or other defects block his personal relations. Homosexuality is essentially psychogenic arising in arrest, disturbance or distortion of psychosexual development in early childhood and crystallized by sixteen years, though studies of identical twins point to a genetic factor. Early seduction is of little consequence in producing homosexual orientation at maturity while parental concern of the consequences are far more damaging to mental development than the seduction per se.

Masturbation with homosexual fantasies is the most frequent homosexual activity while mutual masturbation, bodily contact with interfemoral ejaculations, oral-genital relations, and anal intercourse predominate. Promiscuity is marked among unstable homosexuals, but all homosexuals are more preoccupied with sexual thoughts than heterosexuals. Homosexual acts have a totally different significance in different individuals; the same act may be committed as adolescent experimentation, as the result of mental or physical disorder, or as part of the individual's style of life. The bisexual but predominantly homosexual individual makes some kind of heterosexual adjustment yet desires and seeks homosexual relations. The facultative homosexual is primarily heterosexual but takes part in some homosexual activities under confined circumstances. Finally, there is the psychopathic who partakes of sexual activities as the opportunity arises.

Most homosexuals do not differ in any obvious way from the rest of the population since exhibitionists and feminine pansies are in the minority. They are obsessed with self-condemnation but are driven by logic and psychodynamic forces toward promiscuity with little hope for stable relationships. They remain lonely and alone unable to find someone with whom to share even part of their lives. They are permanent victims of adverse self-definitions imprinted on the sensitive homosexual mind by society. They tend to avoid people and problems by absorption with artistic accomplishments and emotional nuances. Homosexuals are not necessarily bright or gifted with special talents, for many are dullards. Male homosexuals are usually under stress in countries where the law is harsh, but female homosexuals have fewer psychogenic problems because of the more tolerant social and legal attitudes.

Treatment involves change in the direction of the sexual urge to effect greater continence and discretion and above all to achieve better adaptation of the sexual problem in the personal relations of everyday life. The true homosexual rarely undergoes spontaneous resolution. Psychoanalysis offers no hope of cure and endocrine therapy cannot change sexual orientation. The male homosexual who fears to incur social disapproval through lack of control may have his urge reduced or abolished by Stilbesterol 5 to 10 mg daily for physiological castration. Aversion treatment is based on the supposition that homosexuality is a learned reaction which can be unlearned. Mutual discussion about the type of stimuli that tends to incite arousal enables clinical experiments designed for the patient to be exposed to such stimuli while subjected to unpleasant concomitant stimuli simultaneously, such as electric shock, which may cause them to associate with displeasure what was previously pleasurable. Transitional homosexuality is amenable to open discussion holding out the hope even for true homosexuals of a change in sexual orientation, provided the patient seeks opportunities for heterosexual arousals.

Gender Deviations

Development of male sexuality is determined by the boy's ability to manage the fantasied dangers and pleasures of having a penis. His growing awareness of its value as a source of physical pleasure is threatened by his immature fear that he may be deprived of the organ. As an infant he became increasingly aware of his penis by sensing its presence and later by endowing it with meaning. Phallic awareness began long before the actual phallic stage and gave the sense of maleness with membership in the male sex permanently fixed, a sense different from that of masculinity. The one is a matter of identity while the other gradually emerges by experiencing masculinity. The sense of gender identity is thus derived from the awareness of the genitalia, the attitude of parents, siblings, and peers towards his gender role, and the biological force that modifies the environmental roles. A boy may be born without a penis yet mature with a good sense of maleness. The tendency to transform such a male into a female is not possible because of the boy's male behavior characteristics. Any attempt to construct an adequate penis would be futile because it would not have any sexual function. The only danger is the development of homosexuality for once a boy knows that he is a male, he creates a penis that functions symbolically in the same manner as that of the boy with a normal penis.

Development of female sexuality comes with an awareness of a girl's sex from birth via sensory perception of the genitalia with environmental configuration from parents, siblings and peers. But, there are infants born without a vagina which makes a female question her femininity. She may be dubious about the surgical vaginal plastic but never thinks she is a male and never wishes to be converted into a male. Indeed, at maturity the woman with an artificial vagina and an inner mucosa created by a skin graft develops orgasms physiologically indistinguishable from the normal woman. A sense of being a female develops out of the same roots as that of being a male and persists as unalterably in the female as in the male. We cannot consider the clitoris a small penis, masculine, and more active than the vagina, though it has a phallic meaning to a woman because the sense of being a female and feeling feminine is independent of the female genitalia. Such pseudopsychosis or even brain disease does not loosen the core of gender identity. There may be unguarded moments that stir feelings for becoming the opposite sex but the woman still knows her own sex and sticks to it. The vagina is sensed and not eroticized in young girls but the source of their femininity appears long before the oedipic phase emerges during the first year of life.

Male Transsexuality

An apparently normal boy without any biological sex abnormalities develops aberrant psychological variables that distort gender identity. He considers himself trapped in the wrong body with the wrong sex and longs to become a female. Normally, gender identity is less intense, more secret and rather unconscious, but such an unfortunate is confused in his personal sense of identity. Transsexualism is the personal conviction of a biological normal male of being a member of the opposite sex which inevitably leads to requests for endocrinological and surgical procedures in adult years to produce the necessary anatomical changes. The boy is born anatomically male with normal chromosomes and normal XY chromosomes. Nevertheless, he may dress in female clothes or improvise them with appropriate acessories to play the female role in everyday life, develop the gait, posture, gestures, voice inflections of the female, once the feminine role is assumed in dress. He plays exclusively with girls, takes girls' parts in daily life, and even sits to urinate. The mother usually considers it a cute behavior, manifest for brief periods every day, until it becomes a blatant preoccupation in thought, feeling and deed.

Cross-dressing activates psychosexual reidentification. The boy identifies himself with the mother and hates his father. She holds him up against her physically as often as possible, practices excessive intimacy in the nude beyond the normal transient periods of personal relationships. The problem is usually how he is held and for how long he is held, and the feeling of overflowing love in the day and night personal encounters. Every sensation a mother produces upon her boy's body is pleasurable or tension-producing, normal during the first months of life but an emotional aberration for both thereafter. Everything she does and says is in terms of "we" as a couple, whether it be at the table, in the bath or lavatory. The mother's role in boyhood trans-sexuality involves deep-seated unconscious wishes. She is usually a strong bisexual woman with marked penis envy derived from her father, but married to a weak, colorless man.

The son becomes the phallus of her flesh kept as a part of herself and effeminized by identification. Her inability to help her boy separate from her physically reflects her need for him to divest her of the emptiness she received from her own mother. If the boy's father fails to put an end to this couple devouring each other's gender, the boy remains effeminate, develops unusual artistic ability and feminine identification to produce artistic creations. The latent transsexual is intelligent, creative, able to establish warm relationships with both sexes of peers and elders. The feeling that he is assigned to the wrong sex is wrong, but it is not a delusion. The boy's belief is based on prolonged exposure to his mother's body and her attitude in so gratifying a manner as to prolong innate identification with her. Treatment is based on individual assessment, counseling and psychoanalysis. Stilbesterol may control intensive urges at the risk of feminization.

Transvestitism is a disturbance of sex life associated with dress: clothing fetishism with garments of the opposite sex provoking erotic behavior for masturbation; in pseudotransvestitism with a particular type of clothing, not that of the opposite sex, indispensable for sexual experience; in true transvestitism with a tendency to wear clothing of the opposite sex; in male transsexualism with a burning desire for a body configuration of that of the female. Transvestitism represents a crippling form of sex development with hereditary proneness to nervous attitudes but no direct relationship to biological intersexuality, whether the concern is with clothing or body configuration of the opposite sex, or whether it is the wish to maintain his own sex or change with rejection of his own bodily sexuality.

The evolution of the disorder depends on an immature personality secretly practicing his peculiarities under the cover of social and conjugal functions. There may be a deep-seated feeling despite all physical or genetic evidence to the contrary, that he is inherently of the opposite sex. The answer may be difficult for it involves distinguishing between chromosomal, gonadal, hormonal and morphologic sexuality in addition to the sex role assigned by his rearing environment; the one he currently plays, and the one he really feels. The homosexual component is dominant; there is no inner peace until the sex is changed by surgery, mammoplasty and estrogen therapy.

Transsexualism is a deep-seated desire to be transformed into the opposite sex in adolescent males without chromosomal abnormality, who wish to become women and live as such, and in adolescent girls who wish to become men. Each complains that they are spiritually imprisoned in a body of their own sex causing marked frustration in self-expression and self-fulfillment. They are not content with mere adoption of the opposite sexual roles and are not satisfied with anything short of an actual physical change. The transsexualite is unstable and exhibitionistic but not psychotic. He is desperately sincere to the point of attempting suicide if bilateral orchidectomy does not effect the sex change. Surgery involves conservative operative procedures with investigational rather than actual removal of the penis and testes in case of subsequent change of mind. The patient should be required to spend a substantial preoperative trial period supporting himself or herself in the sexual role to which he or she wishes to change.

SEXUAL MATURATION

Youth is a creature of diffuse sexuality. And sex is a mighty but unstable force to be discovered, understood and directed to creative ends for attaining maturity. To become all one can as man or woman requires a growing insight into one's own sexuality and the natural freedom to fulfill it responsibly in genitality. It means understanding of one's self as a sexual being not only when one experiences sexual desires but in everything one does as a man or woman. It has an everyday-ness and an everyplace-ness that affects all relationships, viewpoints, opportunities for fulfillment in every phase of life. Sex is a powerful drive; sex energy is more powerful than nuclear energy. Sex drive and sex behavior are as essential as the correct structure and function of the sex organs, mediated by the neural structure of the brain and the tuned orchestra of hormones. It takes a relatively mature personality to achieve adequate sex relations. The all or none principle maintains in sex, for the slightest deviation to personality structure or function detracts from the effectiveness of the sexual performance. The more mature the adolescent, the more charming; the less mature, the more tedious the youth. Charm is the quality of mature personality that makes the partner more satisfied with himself or herself. And, sex is the great amateur art that reaches up into the ultimate pinnacle of the adolescent spirit as the prime mover of all that he does and is and dreams.

The immature youth bears many a deficiency in total personality to deprive him of the power to grow and mature, for the process of maturing is an art to be learned, an effort to be sustained. But he must have the wherewithal to find the seriousness he had as a child at play. How do we know that the fruit is ripe? Simply because it leaves the branch. After all, to be an adult is to be alone, to live with fear and not be afraid, with the necessary and sufficient fulfillment of his individual SOS, S for sexuality, O for occupation, S for sociality. It is surprising that so many remain profoundly ignorant of the facts of life in this sophisticated age when the sexes mix with so much freedom. The major revolution in the sex behavior in women, made possible by modern contraceptives, led to the adjustment of man to the new concept which women have of themselves in their relationships with men and society. The religious idea that life is a vale of tears is just as false as the idea that life is a field of entertainment. Life is a place of service, and in that service one has to suffer at times a great deal that is hard to bear, and occasionally to experience a great deal of joy. But that joy can only be real if people look upon their life as a service and have a definite object outside themselves and their personal happiness.

Sexual Development

Adolescence and sex are synonymous to parents because the reproductive organs undergo rapid development simultaneously with the marked increase in body height. Enlargement of the external genitalia in boys and onset of the menarche in girls are clinical criteria for establishing not only the beginning but the degree of puberal development, despite wide variations in the time of onset, rapidity of change and completion of development. The stimulus for puberty comes from within the CNS and gonadotropin secretion precedes testicular or ovarian development and secretion. CNS and hypothalamus trigger the puberal timetable. Small amounts of gonadotropin are present before puberty for the development and maintenance of the gonads during this quiescent latent stage; and the prepuberal gonads secrete a small amount of androgen in the male and estrogen in the female. The prepuberal child thus lacks the proper stimulus to gonadotropin release if the pituitary and gonads are not functioning normally. FSH and LH depend on hypothalamic stimulation for their secretion as opposed to the lesser degrees of dependence of ACTH and TSH. Gonadotropin release is inhibited by the traces of androgen or estrogen secreted by the prepuberal gonad. As CNS and anterior hypothalamus become less sensitive to sex hormone, larger amounts of hypothalamic-releasing factors flow to the pituitary and more FSH and LH are released. Sex hormone production is increased to high levels to create the biologic effects of puberty.

TABLE VII

BOYS' SEXUALITY

Childhood (0-10)	Testes and penis show no growth or pubic hair.
Early Adolescence (10-15)	Testes increase in size; scrotum grows, skin reddens and coarsens; penis grows in length and circumference; down but no pubic hair.
Mid-adolescence (11-18)	Pubic hair—pigmented, coarse and straight at base of penis becoming curled and profuse, forming an inverse triangle that extends to umbilicus; axillary hair starts after pubic hair; penis and testes continue growing; scrotum becomes larger, pigmented and sculptured; prostate and seminal vesicles mature; emissions follow; spermatozoa inadequate in number and motility; voice changes as larynx enlarges.
Late Adolescence (14-20)	Facial and body hair spread; pubic and axillary hair densen; voice deepens; testes and penis continue to grow; emission has motile spermatozoa for fertility; indentation of frontal hair line.
Post-adolescence (16-21)	Mature—full development of primary and secondary sex characteristics; musculature and hirsuitism increase.

The first sign of puberal change in boys is enlargement of the scrotum and testes. Testicular growth reflects the growth of the lumina in seminal tubules. Later, Sertoli cells appear, spermatogenia multiply to form the bulk of the testes which initiate spermatogenesis. The testicles and scrotum enlarge and assume a different color and texture. The penis lengthens and a slight growth of long, straight, pigmented hair appears at the base. During the next year, there is further growth of the testes, scrotum and penis, the pubic hair becomes dark and coarse and curls slightly. Two years later, the scrotum becomes darker and larger to contain the bigger testicles, the penis lengthens and broadens and the glans enlarge to adult size. Pubic hair becomes thicker and curly as in the adult until final hair growth indicates cessation of development.

Girls reveal parallel developmental stages. Changes in the breasts and growth of pubic hair are indicators of sexual maturation. Pubic hair first grows along the medial edge of the labia and as in boys it is usually straight, long and slightly pigmented except in members of darker races. During the next year, the hair becomes more abundant, spreads over the labia and pubic areas, becomes pigmented and begins to curl. Further growth leads to the adult pattern; the hair becomes thickest, curls and covers a larger area. Final hair growth as in males involves the medial aspects of the thighs. Breast changes in girls occur in similar stages: first, growth is seen as a small mound with enlargement of the areola and no separation until the areola and nipple form a second mound above the breast. In the final stage the areola becomes part of the breast contour and only the nipple projects.

Developmental stages have diagnostic significance for detecting immaturity in the making in boys and girls. To characterize an adolescent as having a height and weight at a particular age is meaningless in the maturation profile but to observe and record the maturation stages of adolescents is significant data. The time of onset of the growth spurt varies with each individual as do the velocity and time of completion. Participation in contact sports should be based on maturation stage, not on age or weight. It is grossly disadvantageous in sports for a boy in the first stage to compete with one in the final stage, regardless of age and weight. Knowledge of the normal stages alerts the physician to disorders in maturation which serve as an indication for corrective therapy and psychological counseling.

TABLE VIII

GIRLS' SEXUALITY

Childhood (0-9)	Breasts flat; no pubic hair.
Early Adolescence (9-14)	Rounding of hips; breasts and nipples elevated, down but no pubic hair.
Mid-adolescence (10-16)	Pubic hair—pigmented, coarse straight along labia, progressively curled, spreads over mons in an inverse triangular pattern; axillary hair starts after pubic hair. Menarche—labia enlarged; vaginal secretion acid; breasts —areola and nipples elevated.
Late Adolescence (13-18)	Axillary and pubic hair develop; breasts of adult configuration; menstruation established.
Post-adolescence (15-19)	Axillary hair increased; breasts developed.

Psychosexual Development

The thoughts and feelings of the adolescent stirred by sudden changes in shape and size and by new mental abilities and sexual proclivities are far more disturbing than the external influences directed towards him by parents, peers and society. Sexual development is the real criterion of growth and maturity for the anxious adolescent; and secondary characteristics are the biologic basis of attraction between the sexes. The boy compares the features of his body with those of his peers, with respect to height, shoulder breadth, muscle strength, hip narrowness and sexual organs. The girl is equally aware of her changing configuration and compares social acceptance, standards of appearance, weight and shape, because rapid growth in height or weight becomes a source of concern or depression. Boys resort to athletic supports and girls to brassieres to support the ego but a small genitalia and no menarche inhibit youth from mixed group activities.

Sociality first emerges in a strong relationship with a member of the same sex following acceptance by a suitable peer group. Boys brag about the extent of their sexual information, usually erroneous, while girls exaggerate their personal problems. Both sexes gradually become more interested in themselves with remote concern about heterosexual affairs. Boys masturbate in the peer group without acknowledging it to parents. Girls masturbate less than boys but develop a greater sense of guilt. Menstruation is usually welcome even though it may be a distressing experience. More disturbing is the belated occurrence of menstruation up to sixteen or even to eighteen years which usually parallels the failure to be accepted by the peer group.

Youth gradually develops interest in the opposite sex at a distance by notes and phones until dating begins in group functions. Girls prefer to associate with older boys because of earlier maturation. Sex curiosity precludes heterosexual experimentation because of the need to prove one's self sexually, first physically, then emotionally. Early adolescence may involve homosexual relationships until successful coital experiences prove to the boy that he is not a homosexual. But repetition of this pleasurable experience may be marred by fear of pregnancy rather than venereal infection; and so he turns to contraceptives or masturbation to relieve sexual tensions. Apparently, dominating bodies are given youth only to be denied at every turn and their nature is always wrong and wicked; how ineffectual they must feel— like fish not meant to swim. They doubt their sexual effectiveness in the social world; most young men seem to be afraid that they will not be men enough and young women, that they might be considered only women.

TABLE IX

SEXUAL CHARACTERISTICS IN AMERICAN GIRLS

Pelvis:	8-10 years	Female contour and fat deposition.
Breasts:	9-11 years	First hypertrophy or budding.
	12-13 years	Enlargement and pigmentation of nipple.
	16-18 years	Histologic maturity.
Vagina:	11-14 years	Secretion begins, glycogen content increases, changes in cell type.
Pubic hair:	10-12 years	Initial appearance.
	11-15 years	Abundant and curly.
Axillary hair:	12-14 years	Initial appearance.

Maleness and Femaleness

Nature produces no absolute male or absolute female by the very nature of the origin of sex. Somehow, there is something feminine in the virile man and something masculine in the feminine girl. But extremes in either create the third sex. Aren't two sexes enough? Sexual identification involves the incorporation of an outside person of the same sex with one's self. The task is facilitated when the model is admirable, approachable and accepting. It is a learned reaction between the abstraction of the male and female, on the one hand, and certain attitudes and behaviors, on the other. An adolescent boy acquires a conviction that he feels a certain way and does a certain thing, the name

of the game is being masculine, to become a man. It has high
stakes in terms of emotional well-being, vocational options and
personal affiliations. The adolescent process of sexual identification is linked with social factors that strengthen one's sexuality.
Boys tend to band together, foster their automatonism in a common stand against the parents as a show of masculine mastery.
Girls use their peers to develop intimate affiliations in social relations.

Sexual identity is at the core of adolescent identity. Boys with
strong masculine feelings develop good mental health. Girls
with weak feminine orientation are less poised socially with adults
and less socially energetic. Boys consider personal appearance
and achievements in the self-concept while girls view interpersonal attractiveness and popularity crucial in their lives. Sexuality
is influenced by character strivings inherent in the personality
structure and disturbed by character distortions. A sexual relationship becomes a means of seeking out security, expression,
dependency, reassurance, and enhancing or devaluating the self.
Security demanded by self-subjugation means self-annihilation
but security achieved by power striving enables establishment
of dominance over others via the sexual drive.

The specific traits of maleness and femaleness arise from deep-
seated embryonic anlages. The effeminate male is more interested in feminine activities than in masculine. He prefers to
help his mother around the house, has few male friends, and plays
with girls asexually. He has no athletic prowess, appears physically obese and soft. It may be due to a punitive father who is
intolerant of any aggression in his son. He turns to passivity because of the danger of normal aggressiveness, aggravated by a
seductive mother or absence of masculine influence in the home.
The masculine girl suppresses the feminine role, denies or rejects the significance of menstruation. She tends to emulate masculine activities and attire. Tomboyishness in the puberal period abounds in some because of envy of the masculine role; in
others, to establish early male relationships. It is up to the parents to inculcate the gender role throughout childhood before

such identification becomes a social problem. The male-ish girl debates the wisdom of femininity, considers it unsatisfying compared to masculinity. She then proceeds to prove that she is as good or better than boys in all boyish activities. The pattern may persist unto adult life and naturally leads to lesbian adjustment. A daughter of a domineering, unfeminine mother identifies with her and grows up accordingly. Another adolescent girl reared in a home situation where the mother is masochistic deplores the degradation by a sadistic father. The daughter considers it unpleasant to become a woman like her mother, wants to be more like her father and identifies with his type, becomes aggressive, and marries a passive man whom she dominates.

Deviation from nature is deviation from happiness. Nature takes no account of even the most reasonable of human excuses. Grown up, it's a terribly hard thing to maintain. It is much easier to skip it and go from one childhood to another. But the civilized adolescent cannot fully satisfy his sexual instinct without normal sexual love. Sex is the great amateur art to be mastered. Athena sprang forth from the head of Zeus but humans attain adult sexuality through an unfolding sequence of interpersonal, biological and psychological stages of artful techniques modified by parents, peers and the world at large. The adolescent, in particular, needs help in understanding the reproductive process and in mastering his own feelings and impulses. Sex information corrects misconceptions to establish sexuality at the individual norm. The measure of healthy sexual behavior is the capacity to realize creative potentials and live up to responsibilities in order to live in harmony with others. The function of sex goes beyond procreation as a determining factor in the growth of character, maturity of emotions and evolutions of personality. It is something youth cannot comprehend for the appetite for sex seems like the appetite for food. A young man can enjoy his dinner all alone at the table but he needs a partner to enjoy sex, and if he masturbates, he has an imaginary partner for the sexual act as the supreme expression of an interpersonal relationship.

TABLE X

MALE GONADAL EVALUATIONS

Physical Examination

FSH-dependent development—Increase in testicular size

LH and testosterone-dependent development
Temporal hair recession
Beard growth
Voice change
Penis and prostate growth

Laboratory Tests
Buccal smear
Karyotype
Bone age

Endocrine Evaluation

Hypothalamic-pituitary function
LH and FSH secretion
Clomiphene stimulation test
Growth hormone, ACTH, TSH secretion

Leydig cell function
Testosterone secretion
HCG stimulation test

Seminiferous tubule function
Semen analysis
Testicular biopsy

Sexual Relationship

Childish love knows no bounds; it demands exclusive possession and is satisfied with nothing less than all. But it has a
second characteristic; it has no real aim, being incapable of
complete satisfaction in returning the parental love, hence doomed
to end in disappointment and to give place to a hostile attitude.
But a well-mated couple are as eager to give sexual satisfaction
as to receive it. They grow to appreciate the aphorism that it
is more blessed to give than to receive in learning each other's
sex needs and in perfecting their sexual skills. The couple reach
maturity when they have achieved an harmonious sexual relationship devoted to giving satisfaction. The summit of their sex
potentialities is reached when the quest for an orgasm is not the
satisfaction to get for one's self, but to give to one's partner.

The higher values of sex promote growth of character and fulfillment of responsibility. A personal philosophy based on any-

thing less than this high purpose degrades sex in our era of sexual freedom. When adolescents engage in free love they deceive themselves to think that they are free. They use sex as a low channel for neurotic urges not in the service of its higher purpose. A young man will seduce one girl after another with no feeling of love or commitment but only to prove his manhood; but a man who is sure of his manhood is under no compulsion to prove it. A girl may have a succession of affairs to assure herself that she is attractive to men or in the belief that it is the best way to get a husband. There is no dearth of young men who will accept her free favors and so she invariably suffers a blow to her self-esteem.

These adolescents consider themselves free but they are free only of the burdens of social responsibility and slaves to their neurotic compulsions. Fun morality desecrates every society. Sexual behavior is mature and healthy when geared to the highest level of responsibility, when sexuality is the vehicle for the expression of maximal love, tenderness and devotion. But it is immature and unhealthy when it serves self-indulgence, exploitation or satisfaction of neurotic needs. The affirmation of one's life, growth and freedom is rooted in one's capacity to love with respect and responsibility. If youth is able to love productively, he loves himself too; if he can only love others, he cannot love at all. The adolescent must achieve the degree of sex fulfillment necessary and sufficient for body metabolism and mental health, otherwise he suffers frustration and failure, compromises with neurosis or psychosis, or retreats to disease or degeneration. Sexuality in the making determines the pattern of personality, the caliber of occupation planning, the level of sociality, the effectiveness of interrelationship. Each of these developmental processes proceeds at its own tempo revealing innate potentialities, home rearing, peer influence, school guidance and heterogeneous effects that tend to merge into harmonious or discordant maturation. Developmental accretions reach geometric not arithmetic proportions in the dynamic life of youth.

The idealized concept of sexual relationship ignores the wide gap between romantic love and mundane realities. The varied forms and wide ranges of normal sexual behavior are adaptations of the sex impulse to the social setting. The physiology of sex provides a very incomplete account of the pervasive importance of the sexual instinct in the development and fulfillment of adolescent personality. The ability to create and sustain an unselfish relationship with a member of the opposite sex is but one valid measure of emotional maturity since man and woman united make the complete human being. The spontaneous expression of the sexual instinct is modified by social, economic, religious and cultural forces, acting in different ways in different societies. The diversity of human sexuality is the most remarkable feature despite stylized versions of the sexual relationship which give little account of the varied forms which sexual behavior may assume. The dominant instinct so essential to the survival of the species is one of the mainsprings of human motivation, and the fulfillment or frustration is closely bound up with adolescent happiness or misery.

Adolescents pass a phase of homosexual interest, especially in single-sex boarding schools, continuing through part or all of adult life with a sexual orientation of this type. The distinction between a hetero or homosexual interest is not absolute with ambivalent dispositions for an individual may be capable of enjoying sexual outlets of both types. It is thus difficult to classify people as either homosexuals or heterosexuals, hence estimates of the frequency of homosexuality in Western societies range from 1:7 to 1:50. But early recognition of deviant behavior as the way of youth calls for discrete guidance and/or professional participation in the desired libido objective. Sex is not only what one looks like but what one does. Every adolescent must be positive about accepting his or her sex to cultivate the optimal in the bond-to-be for emotional stability. The adolescent male has sexual fantasies, diurnal erections, nocturnal seminal ejaculations and erotic dreams. Infants, impotent and satiated males also develop erections during sleep. Voluntary relief from sexual tension may be achieved by masturbation. It is not physically harmful, but if an individual feels guilty or anxious about its supposed effects, the conflict between these feelings and the compulsion to seek such a sexual outlet may become emotionally disruptive.

Adolescence is a stage between childhood and adultery. Youth develops intermittent sexual frustration enhanced by the cinema, radio, television, fashion, advertising, pornography and publishing. The authority of parental, ecclesiastical or school injunctions is ignored. Petting abounds with intimate physical contacts to increase the intensity of erotic arousal, stopping short of coitus, but culminating in orgasm. Many adolescents are unable or unwilling to accept the restraint involved in petting and have premarital intercourse with the protection of the pill or other devices or nothing. Blatant intercourse is more common among those of lower social class who marry at an earlier age with conception preceding marriage. Two-thirds of the women who marry before the age of twenty are pregnant before marriage, hence illegitimate births abound in all races. Premarital intercourse is biologically natural when marriage has to be deferred and emotionally helpful for a marital relationship. Morality in sexual relations, when it is free from superstition, consists essentially of respect for the other person and unwillingness to use that person solely as a means of personal gratification without regard to his or her desires.

The desire to be thought of as experienced and worldly may persuade teenagers to take part in sexual intercourse although they do not really enjoy it. There may be strong pressures upon a boy to prove his masculinity and upon a girl from the fear that she will lose the boy if she does not agree to intercourse. Then, too, there are situations where neither the boy nor the girl really want it, but both feel impelled to participate. Less attractive consequences of premarital intercourse are pregnancy and venereal disease. Among young women, one in three is likely to become pregnant as a result of premarital intercourse. Impregnation may occur without penetration despite coitus interruptus. Reliable methods of contraception are not often compatible with the circumstances of premarital intercourse. Direct transmission of venereal disease can occur with either homosexual or heterosexual contacts.

Youth must develop a degree of maturity to control the carnal excess which leads to impregnation of someone young. Such an experience produces permanent and profound physical, emotional and mental repercussions. The complications of early pregnancy and labor are less than those anticipated in the mature woman, but there are social, legal and genetic problems to confuse the picture. The prevalence of toxemia of pregnancy, especially eclampsia, is probably due to failure of antenatal care until pregnancy is far advanced. There is a high incidence of prematurity but a low incidence of difficult delivery and low fetal loss rate. The age of the mother does not increase the likelihood of abnormal progeny but the increased incidence of prematurity leads to fetal abnormality. The offspring of a close blood relationship between the parents is always susceptible to abnormality caused by recessive genes, for rare recessive defects are invariably increased in consanguinous matings. Incestuous unions encouraged in precocious motherhood increase the possibility of the offspring having a recessive gene abnormality, but in the absence of the family history of such defect, the absolute risk will not be serious though the likelihood of a congenital malformation will be twice that of any random mating.

TABLE XI

DEFICIENT PUBERTY

Boys	*Girls*
Surgical castration	Surgical castration
Developmental delay; generalized debility and chronic illness; congenital or constitutional defects	Developmental multiple congenital or constitutional defects; generalized debility and chronic illness
Generalized hypopituitarism with dwarfism	Generalized hypopituitarism with dwarfism
Specific hypogonadotropinism	Specific hypogonadotropinism
Klinefelter's syndrome	Turner's syndrome
Idiopathic hyporchia or anorchia	
Idiopathic late puberty with tall stature or early puberty with short stature	

Coital Behavior

What is more important in adolescent life than his body or in his world than what youth looks like? If anything is sacred, his human body is sacred. He is endowed with an elaborate, dominating body charged with inner wisdom that seeks full expression in society. If the sex urge is denied at every turn, if his nature is considered wicked, he becomes ineffectual, like a fish not meant to swim. After all, the orgasm has replaced the cross as the focus of longing and the image of fulfillment. When you put a young man and a young woman together, there are some things they simply have to do. They embrace, they warm each other. All the rest leads to lifelong conditioning that may enhance or destroy the joy of sexuality. Normal mating behavior is essential for normal coitus; mating behavior is the effect of gonadal hormones on CNS. In man, libido is determined by testosterone secretion as is sexual activity, and the estrogen secretion of the female partner enhances male sexual activity. In woman, sexual desire is determined by testosterone from the adrenal or ovary, and by estrogen and progesterone. Sexual receptivity to the male tends to be optimal at ovulation and minimal at estrus.

Sexual intercourse involves four distinct phases: excitement, plateau, orgasm and resolution. This step-by-step advancement towards the sexual climax correlates psychoanalytically with the ladders or steps in dreams symbolizing the sexual act as a wish or fear. Experimental studies reveal changes in the shape of the vaginal barrel, corrugation of the vagina, uterine erection or elevation. Normally, the uterus points upward and forward but during coitus it shifts upward and backward with a tenting effect at the vaginal vault where the pool of semen forms. After the female orgasm, the mouth of the uterus gapes, the womb undergoes contraction comparable to the first stage of labor but without the subjective feeling of pain. Oxytocin release induced by genital manipulation causes uterine contraction as an aid to sperm transport. Rhythmic contractions of the uterus and vagina during orgasm are thus associated with rapid passage of sperm into the uterus. The corrugation of the vaginal wall acts as a frictional aid to the penis.

The vaginal environment is highly acid, pH 3.8, while the seminal plasma in which the spermatozoa is dispersed is moderately alkaline, pH 7.3. The acid immobilizes the sperm to hinder its progress but the buffering effect of the seminal plasma neutralizes the acidity. Apparently, the volume of the ejaculate and buffering power are the determining factors in infertility rather than the actual sperm count. Some males would be adjudged fertile by laboratory standards but remain infertile because their spermatozoa are immediately immobilized upon deposition within the vagina. Sexual union may take place at any time, even during menstruation. Desire may be greater in some women at the time of ovulation, in mid-cycle, and just before and after menstruation, but there is no clear-cut cycle of human sexual responsiveness comparable with estrus. However, the physiological phases of the menstrual cycle are accompanied by a pattern of emotional fluctuations, reflected in mood, behavior and dream content. The premenstrual and menstrual parts of the cycle may make the woman more susceptible to scholastic failure, penal offenses and even to suicide.

The female attracts by clothing, cosmetics, coiffure and the male responds with arousal. We may contrast this pattern with that of many species of birds and animals, where the female is dull and frowsy, and sexual display is exclusively the prerogative of the male. The visual stimuli may arouse the male without physical contact but the tactile sensations that arouse the female are the most important in evoking her sexual response. Courtship may begin with touching fingers that bind both spiritually, but it proceeds to more intimate embraces, culminating in the highest degree of epithelial contiguity during coitus. Erogenous zones include the lips in both sexes and the breasts and nipples in women but the glans penis and clitoris are most sensitive. Tactile stimuli from these areas increase the intensity of emotion producing local and bodily changes.

The traditional belief that sexual arousal and response in women are inherently slower than in men was disproven by

Kinsey and Masters. A woman may not become aroused until continuous physical contacts are established because she is less responsive to psychic stimuli. Consequently, the progress of her responses can be arrested by any discontinuity of physical stimulation, and so she may appear highly distractible at a time when the man's excitation is maintained by mental stimuli alone. The response of a female to the point of orgasm during coitus can be no less rapid than that of the male, with uninterrupted physical stimulation. Erection of the penis precedes physical contact and with further stimulation there is elevation and retraction of the testes. The woman's nipples become erect and the breasts hyperemic. The clitoris enlarges and becomes erect; the labia minora shows intense vascular engorgement; and the congested walls of the lower part of the vagina narrow the lumen at this level. The upper vagina becomes elongated due to retraction of parametrial muscle fibers. The greater vestibular glands secrete some mucus but the real lubricant during coitus is a vaginal transudate accompanying the hyperemic changes to allow easy penetration of the penis into the vagina.

The intense sensations resulting from movement of the penis within the vagina culminate in mutual orgasm followed by physical relaxation, mental tranquility and often somnolence. All animals are saddened by the orgasm but human love transcends. With the male orgasm, ejaculation of seminal fluid into the upper vagina takes place; with the female orgasm, irregular reflex contractions of the voluntary muscles investing the vagina persist. In some women, enhanced myometrial contractions occur accompanied by the release of oxytocin. The thrusting movements of the penis within the vagina, in firm contact with the interior vaginal wall, may milk secretions in retrograde fashion along the lumen of the female urethra, and introduce organisms into the bladder with consequent cystitis, occasionally hemorrhagic. During coitus, the pulse rate, blood pressure and pulmonary ventilation are increased. Later, patchy flushing of the skin is often evident, followed by increased sweating. After the male orgasm, erection may rapidly disappear with a refractory period during which further sexual stimulation will evoke no response. There is no refractory phase in women for some may experience orgasms with continuous stimulation in any coital posture: standing, sitting, kneeling or lying.

Heterosexual love is an achievement of the total personality which attains a new level of integration through the adolescent process. Some reach the goal by passing through all phases in a relatively short time; some experience one or more phases only in dreams and fantasies; others pass through one of the stages quickly and may be caught in another for a long delay with struggle. In many cases, the process repeats itself, for regression appears after periodic disappointments, but adolescence ends when the alternatives are narrowed down and youth casts his lot with the chosen modes of sexual activity. The tortuous adolescent process thus involves normal psychopathology in sexual maturation intricately interwoven with personality development in both sexes. But sexual maturation must proceed unabated to transform all hidden potentialities into living realities with a compatible mate. The great objective is the ultimate fusion of a mature male with a mature female into a fruitful bond. The body changes are deep-seated with stimulation of metabolism and mind and stabilization of endocrines and emotions. The sex desire may come in cycles or peaks of activity or desire during any given menstrual cycle for any given couple. The hormonal state of one partner may affect the other to catalyze the understanding which develops between them over the years. It may, indeed, offer a biological explanation for monogomy and the sanctity of marriage in man. The personal entente between the man and woman is durable when the independence is equal, the dependence mutual, and the obligation reciprocal.

I have reason to believe that a man needs something that is more than friendship and is not love, as it is generally understood. This something, nevertheless, only a woman can give. If the heart of a man is depressed with cares, the mist is dispelled when the woman appears. Man can only suffer, while woman can endure. The Book of Life begins with a man and a woman in a garden. It ends with revelations that explain all mysteries except her own. A long courtship is the prelude to constancy of love. Passion strikes root and gathers strength before marriage is grafted on it. Such a union is something you have to give your whole mind to with body and soul, which is a matter of profound wonder. Mozart, inspired by a concert, experienced the feeling that a couple aware of a gradual acquisition of beauty, a marvelous understanding, a sublime reconciliation of conflicting themes are embarked upon one of the few adventures in life—great love, an incomprehensible mingling of friendship, sensuality and respect, without which there is no true marriage.

REFERENCES

Acord, L. D.: Sexual symbolism as a correlate of age. *J. Consult. Psychol.,* *26*:279-281, 1962.

Bell, A. L.: The significance of scrotal sac and testicles for the prepuberty male. *Psychoanal. Qu., 34*:182-206, 1965.

Blank, L. *et al.*: Voyeurism and exhibitionism. *Percept. Mot. Skills, 24*:391-400, 1967.

Bock, E. W. *et al.*: Social status, heterosexual relations and expected ages of marriage. *J. Gen. Psychol., 101*:43-51, 1962.

Donovan, B. T. *et al.*: *Physiology of Puberty.* London, Arnold, 1965.

Dreger, R. M.: Just how far can social change, change personality. *J. Psychology, 64*:167-191, 1966.

Eysenck, H. J.: Personality and sexual adjustment. *Br. J. Psychiatry, 118*: 593-608, 1971.

Farnham, M. F.: Early and late adolescence. *J. Am. Med. Wom. Assoc., 23*:155-8, 1968.

Faust, H. S.: Developmental maturity as a determinant in prestige of adolescent girls. *Child Dev., 31*:173-184, 1960.

Frailberg, S. H.: Homosexual conflicts. In S. Lorand and H. I. Schneer (Eds.): *Adolescents.* New York, Hoeber, 1961.

Gordis, L. *et al.*: Evaluation of a program for preventing adolescent pregnancy. *N. Engl. J. Med., 282*:1078-81, 1970.

Green, R. *et al.*: Effeminacy in prepubertal boys. *Pediatrics, 27*:286-291, 1961.

Hatford, T. C. *et al.*: Personality correlates of masculinity-femininity. *Psychol. Rep., 21*:881-4, 1967.

Harlow, H. *et al.*: Learning to love. *Am. Scientist, 54*:244-272, 1966.

Hemming, J.: *Problems of Adolescent Girls.* London, Heinemann, 1960.

Israel, S. L.: Normal puberty and adolescence. *Ann. N. Y. Acad. Sci., 142*: 773-8, 1967.

Josselyn, I. M.: The capacity to love: a possible reformulation. *J. Am. Acad. Child Psychiatry, 10*:6-22, 1971.

Kinch, R. A.: Adolescent sex-education. *Ann. N. Y. Acad. Sci., 142*:824-33, 1967.

Kirkendall, L. A.: *Understanding Sex.* Life Adjustment Booklet, Chicago, Science Research Associates, 1957.

Marmor, J. (Ed.): *Sexual Inversion.* New York, Basic Books, 1965.

Masters, W. H. *et al.: Human Sexual Inadequacy.* Boston, Little, Brown, 1970.

Masterson, J. Jr.: The old order changeth. *Int. J. Psychiatry, 5*:486-91, 1968.

Mathis, J. L.: The development of sexual identification. *Southern Med. J., 59*:1282-6, 1966.

Mead, B. T.: Masculinity and femininity in our time. *Postgrad. Med., 44*: 244-7, 1968.

Money, J.: *Factors in the Genesis of Homosexuality in Determinants of Human Sexual Behavior.* G. Winokur (Ed.): Springfield, Thomas, 1963; *Sex Errors of the Body.* Baltimore, Johns Hopkins Press, 1968.

Mussen, P. H. *et al.:* The behavior-inferred motivation of late- and early-maturing boys. *Child Dev., 29*:61-67, 1958.

Offer, D. *et al.:* Profiles of normal adolescent girls. *Arch. Gen. Psychiatry, 19*:513-22, 1968.

Osofsky, H. J.: Adolescent sexual behavior. *Clin. Obstet. Gynecol., 14*:393-408, 1971.

Packard, V.: *The Sexual Wilderness.* New York, McKay, 1968.

Schonfeld, W. A.: Adolescence: inappropriate sexual development and body image. *J. Am. Med. Wom. Assoc., 22*:847-55, 1967.

Settlage, C. F.: Adolescence and social change. *J. Am. Acad. Child Psychiatry, 9*(2):203-215, 1970.

Spock, B.: *Teenager's Guide to Life and Love.* New York, Simon & Schuster, 1970.

Stoller, R. J.: The sense of femaleness. *Psychoanal. Q., 37*:42-55, 1968.

Storr, A.: *Sexual Deviation.* Baltimore, Penguin Books, 1964.

Young, W. C. *et al.:* Hormones and sexual behavior. *Science, 143*:212-218, 1964.

Zuger, B.: Effeminate behavior present in boys from early childhood. *J. Pediatr., 68*:1098-107, 1966.

CHAPTER VII

PERSONALITY IMMATURITY

Seek not abroad, turn back into itself
for in the inner man dwells the truth.

Man is a growing animal and his birthright is positive development. His primary adolescence is the spring season between childhood and maturity. It's a process not a product and makes everything seem possible with the soul in ferment, the character undecided, the way of life uncertain, the ambition thick-sighted. The wings of the spirit are still tied down, the love of life immature, the hatred of man premature. We must not be critical of youth's affections, trying on one face after another to find a face of his own. He is so strong, so mad, so certain and so lost; he has everything and is able to use nothing. Yet youth undergoes deep-seated biological, psychological and social changes, emerges at a dramatic rate and unparalleled complexity into manhood or womanhood under genetic, hypothalamic, and environmental forces. They provide the bitter and the sweet of life but the rest of maturity comes from youth's own efforts, with all the abiding traits of character that constitute the potential to respond in special ways to circumstances. Youth thus rides alternately on the horses of his private and public nature to give him the particular stamp of his unique personality.

Deficient Personality

What is more important in the life of the adolescent than his sense of his own uniqueness? His individuation is based on fulfillment of many tasks deficient in optimal functioning of the body machine and of the inner self, with consequent physical, mental, emotional and social inadequacies. The immature are like thistledown blown about by the wind, up and down, here and there, with one in a thousand ever getting beyond seedhood to maturity. In some, the blade springs but does not go on to flower; in others, there is flowering but no fruit is subsequently produced. How do we know that the fruit is ripe? Simply because it leaves the branch. No youth passes that subtle line between childhood and adulthood until he moves from the passive voice of dependence to the active voice of independence. To be adult is to be alone; and to live with fear and not be afraid is the final test of maturity. In the lexicon of youth, which fate reserves for a bright maturity, there is no such word as fail. Yet many fail even though youth is not the creature of circumstance; but circumstance, the creature of youth.

Failure to break parental images precludes building suitable attachments in the maturation process. Saturated bonds wane as unsaturated forces become available. Adolescence involves destruction of early parental images and replacement by current love objects. The impulse to destroy is as nearly universal as the impulse to create—the one is an easier way than the other of demonstrating youth power. Destruction of internal images is either slow or continuous, repetitive or sudden, discontinuous and reparative with accompanying turbulence, if the internalized bonds are not replaced immediately by desired attachments. Adolescent evolution thus involves a constant remodeling of the organism in adaptation to new conditions, but it depends on the nature of those conditions whether the direction of the modifications shall be upward or downward. Developmental deviations occur when the internalized love objects are not given up, but kept inviolate by idealization; or the infantile attachment is so completely withdrawn without replacement that it becomes necessary to regress to pathological self-investment; or finally, the free energy becomes directed towards inappropriate, unrewarding or sadistic objects. If the internalized parental image remains fixed, the adolescent has a Peter Pan look with its appropriate childish behavior and immature physical development. If the infantile attachment to parents is withdrawn completely without replacement, the regression gives the clinical picture of psychosis or severe psychosomatic disorder. If the infant attachment to parents is almost entirely withdrawn, the symptomatology and the resultant depression may lead to suicide. If there be substitution of improper objects, antisocial behavior is inevitable.

Failure to adjust to the loss of love is a terrible thing; they lie who say that death is worse. Youth is never so defenseless against suffering as when they love; never so helplessly unhappy as when they have lost their loved object or its love. What the adolescent knows is everywhere at war with what he wants. He is sure to be a loser when he quarrels with himself; it is an internal civil war in which triumphs are defeats. Youth must not only relinquish his sexual and hostile wishes but loosen all affectionate ties to his parents; this leads to grief aggravated by abandonment of his dependence on the parents. The normal adolescent moodswings resemble the early schizophrenic process, related to self-centeredness from floods of instinctual energies which have been liberated but not yet attached to new individuals. The ego treats the superego as though it were a taboo lover in his struggle for freedom and independence; it rebels against submission to an authority from without or from within. The adolescent's need to reorient himself to new object relations after withdrawing energies from early ones involves a struggle to maintain contact with being too close, a struggle to be independent while hating them, and a struggle to discharge sexual tension even through fantasy. The rapid shifts in adolescent "crushes" are necessary escapes from primary love objects. When in love, youth is manic-elated; when out of love, morose-depressed; and between loves, the feelings of inner loss are so intense as to become depersonalized. The hostility and aggression which serve as defenses against object love soon become intolerable and aggression may be turned away from the object inwardly against the self, with consequent depression, self-abasement, and self-injury that may lead to suicide.

Failure to become an independent being is due to inadequate emotional independence. There is conflict between the adolescent's urgent demands for emancipation and the parents' attempt to enforce restrictions. There is insistent but feeble demand for privacy, with complete dissociation from parents and elders. Obviously, the immature adolescent fails to achieve the initial stage of individuation; he fails to develop identity because of an unstable self-concept. Normally, the adolescent develops an accurate idea about himself embodying both physical and psychological self-image of his strengths and weaknesses, expectations and promises from society, facts and foibles about the sexual role, schemes and dreams of a full life plan. Every attempt to put plans into action creates conflict between adolescent and adult about the ineptness of the endeavors: altruistic one moment and self-centered the next; perceptive one time and obtuse the next; prejudiced and tolerant on the same issue; shifting occupational aspirations; vacillating between childish and mature behavior; veering from one philosophical commitment to another; arguing for asceticism while glorying in luxury; chasing women while extolling monastic life, all with feeling, passion and purpose. Emotional instability of the normal adolescent is seen in much lesser disguise in the immature adolescent who sees nothing because he knows nothing.

Failure of self-motivation deprives the immature youth of initiative and direction. He is not free but shows increasing resistance to act when adults direct his behavior. But with more responsibility gained, more self-reliance is established; he begins to scratch his head with his own nails. An immature adolescent behaves like a young child responding relatively well to direct requests in contradiction to the normal adolescent who resents adult guidance. Failure to establish appropriate values for adult behavior excludes him from practicing the ethical system of his community. The immature adolescent does not exhibit the kind of behavior conducive to passionate, personal attachments and for group relationships in mastering the philosophical principles of life. He has no notion of conscience, no relish for virtue, no moral restraints from hope or fear. Failure of empathy for anybody precludes any form of reciprocity for interpersonal relationships. The normal adolescent cultivates the ability to respect others and gain his own ends without trampling upon others' rights. He appreciates human beings as individuals not as objects to satisfy or block his needs. He interprets other people's actions and attempts to understand them through a process of mutual exploration, abstract probings not discerned in immature youth.

Failure to establish appropriate sexual identity prevents acceptance of one's self as a sexually mature being and thus blocks development of meaningful heterosexual relationships. The normal adolescent accepts his changed adult body and mature sexuality, while the immature youth is unprepared to adapt to such adult roles. Youth always wishes to change something about him—his complexion, weight, height, facial features, body proportions, teeth or almost anything to achieve "perfection." There is a compelling preoccupation with physical appearance, sexual features and wearing apparel for simulating physical sameness with peers. There is rumination about physical normality and concern about late sexual development. The initial sexual outlet is sexual masturbation in both male and female; it extends to sexual experiences with others of the same sex, and finally to heterosexual activities. Youth wanders, but in the end there is always a peace of mind in being what he is, in being that completely; this is the first step toward becoming better than he is. The difference between generations is that parents ask what have we experienced? And adolescents, what can we experience? Youth cannot create experience; youth must undergo it; and that is difficult, if not impossible for the immature who misuses life at every turn. The hardest thing to cope with is not selfishness or vanity or deceitfulness, but immaturity.

Failure to develop new intellectual capacities indicates lack of mental acceleration during early adolescence. Youth first becomes capable of abstract thinking with change in perceptions of time and space, with differentiation of past from future. But the immature adolescent rarely reaches the full intellectual potential by age sixteen. Failure to function satisfactorily with age blocks appropriate behavior with peer groups. Good achievement in this area is an important index of the caliber of adolescent development, correlating with good achievement in other tasks. Most adolescents conform, for nonconformists are rejected and ridiculed. Adolescents have become a significant subculture with their dress, language, music and values, all somewhat denied the immature adolescent. Failure to develop moral values during adolescence is partly due to lack of ability to reason abstractly.

Youth must reform values and make them his own as part of his emancipation from parents. It is part of the need to develop broader, more flexible moral concepts rather than merely re-ordering childhood rules of behavior. He is likely to become aware of the large gaps between the things people tell him to do and the things they actually do themselves. For once, he perceives that his parents have more weakness than strength and develops a sense of outrage over the gulf between social idealism and social practices in the light of current upheavals to our society. But the immature youth is totally oblivious of this state of affairs.

Failure to control aggressive impulses is a major moral concern. All impulse manages everything badly. Youth may shift from being active sexually to refraining from sexual activity. He may replace rage, fury and violence with peaceful self-restraint and saint-like gentleness, as normal aspects of adolescence to which impulsive activity and excessive self-control swing back and forth, in ever-narrowing cycles. This leads to slow development of the ability to acquire realistic controls over himself and to release feelings without guilt or anxiety. Adolescents living in families with democratic rather than authoritarian self-government are able to control behavior without becoming overly inhibited, becoming self-reliant, poised and effective ever free to criticize parents in friendly companionship. But, adolescents of authoritarian parents are obedient on the surface and rebellious beneath this facade, with an externalized morality that is quite transparent. Youth must aim above morality; he must not be simply good, but good for something despite the legal status of a minor by reason of immaturity. He must be protected by the power of the state from his lack of judgment and from unjust overreaching by others. The science of legislation is like that of medicine in that it is far more easy to point out what will do harm than what will do good. Fragile as reason is, and limited as law is as the institutionalized medium of reason, that's all we have standing between us and the tyranny of mere will and the cruelty of un-bridled, undisciplined adolescent feeling.

Failure to develop purpose in life reduces youth to the life of a spider in suspense. The immature adolescent discloses an endless search for purpose but he is never able to sustain any constructive activity at home, in school, with playmates or with hobbies to a point of gratification, despite intentions. It is not a question of not having purpose but in not being able to feel a sense of purpose in life. And, lack of purpose represents a distortion in identification. An ideal purpose in life is a highly exaggerated concept with false implications. Living in a society in which youth is constantly exhorted to think big and act big, they have attached this same bigness to purpose. It represents an attempt at grasping life in a grandiose futuristic manner and so each disregards the now in his existence. Sometimes it is difficult to deal with this megalomaniac resistance to turn the adolescent to the minute by minute presence of his fast moving life. By accentuating now, he does what he can do to accomplish the purpose of being himself. By not accepting now, but dreaming of a purpose, he carries out the infantile continuity of his father and hopes to share in his anticipation. After all, purpose in life is being one's self in life and not being somebody else's self. Man cannot approach the Divine by reaching beyond the human; he can approach Him by becoming human.

DEFECTIVE PERSONALITY

Most personality problems either involve development or adjustment; developmental problems are normal variations in behavior that are a phase of growing up and will usually pass if not mishandled; adjustment reactions are temporary personality difficulties that arise from transitional situations, environmental pressures, or from adolescent problems in coping with increased instinctual strivings. Apart from these, there are chemical mental diseases, psychotic personality disorders, neuroses and psychosomatic illnesses. We must distinguish developmental and adjustment problems from emotional derangements; the former are minor and transient and the latter, major and prolonged. Diagnostic difficulties arise because the normal adolescent shows moodiness, sensitiveness, irritability, often confused with withdrawal behavior unto a schizophrenic world. The adolescent presents bizarre manifestations because the image of himself which he tries to create in his own mind, in order that he may love himself, is very different from that which he tries to create in the minds of others in order that they may love him.

Personality profile is self-revealing: the multiple face, the biographer; the total physique, the recorder; the deviant behavior, the revealer. Every case smells of the wine it contains. Knowledge of the adolescent personality must not remain inert like a crystal ball on the desk. The youth who repeatedly finds himself at odds with the environment may finally come around to wonder what is wrong. Patient and physician can be completely candid to make a correct diagnosis, interpret the life style and formulate the remedial therapy. The personality type is clearly demonstrated by youth's sexual behavior: the obsessive type will be orderly, obstinate and miserly in every phase of his relationship; the schizoid will neither give nor take; the paranoid will look for someone to blame. Yet every youth can be encouraged to try more mature ways of reacting to counter his inner tendencies. And the first sign of improvement in any personality disorder will be the recognition of another person's needs and not just his own. Adolescent character is formed in the stream of human life.

Sex and sex differences unravel distinct personality patterns. The maturity tasks of both sexes are the same but the style of solving them is quite different. A young woman accepts the limitations of reality more readily than a man, but in doing so she must come to terms with her conflicting wishes. Her passive side demands intimacy and the presence of someone to love; her more active side demands gratification through mastery without masculine emphasis in competition. She must achieve a balance between being and doing, pleasing and being pleased, submitting and resisting, wishing and acting since imbalance leads to deep-seated depression. A young man, on the other hand, accepts the limitations of reality less readily. He tries to modify the external world rather than be modified himself. He emphasizes action and mastery and restricts competition to safe areas such as sports. Any failure to adapt will manifest itself by a change in activity rather than in mood. And the male reaction to any threat to self-esteem is apathy rather than depressive feelings.

The apathetic male substitutes passive for active aims to protect his self-esteem depleted by loss or threatened by fears that activity will lead to injury. He accepts the passive feeling of being able to modify reality by pretending the effort is not important. He has not lost; he has decided not to act. He protects himself by saying, "I could do it now if I wished to and I will someday." Inner life is idealized at the expense of outer life, hence some adolescents resort to drug abuse; others drop out to search for a nonthreatening outer reality; still others substitute idealized passive protest in place of active rebellion. Most adolescents become active again when satisfying life experiences with adults ameliorate the long-felt threat to self-esteem.

Personality forces develop throughout adolescence, hence the difficulty of inferring an apparent abnormality as a settled feature of youth's makeup. The unstable, impulsive, aggressive adolescent tends to become more stable with maturation as cerebral dysrhythmias become normal. The psychopathic is the end-product of deprivation; he must make society either acknowledge deprivation of a loved object or provide a satisfactory structure to withstand the strains of his spontaneous movements. The neurotic, phobic youth bedeviled by unconscious motivation may show marked inadequate traits that tend to persist to maturity. The eccentric youth preoccupied with esoteric pursuits may become a misfit in the world yet cannot be considered schizoid. Change of environment or response to treatment may determine the future status of his personality with a stable sense of identity. The schizophrenic cannot feel real in all phases of life yet may achieve something on the basis of living by proxy. The paranoid is dominated by a system of thought that rationalizes constantly to explain everything, else there is acute confusion of ideas, sense of chaos and loss of predictability.

The personality profile of the mental, emotional and social behavior determines whether the mental state is a causation of illness in its own right or a reaction of the immature personality to his experiences. Immature adolescents may not suffer from any definite mental or emotional disorder yet reveal psychiatric problems. The term psychopathic personality embodies too much to be meaningful. It is a question of neurotic acting out vs. neurotic symptoms. The presence of an unconscious neurotic conflict can easily be recognized from the irrationality of behavior, from stereotyped repetitive acting out of unconscious motive, from distortion of unconscious fantasies. Abnormal adolescent personalities embody a whole range of neurotic disorders, such as anxiety neurosis, endogenous depression, hysteria and obsessional neurosis. They can occur singly or in combinations from a crushing blow or from marked anxiety for there is something of hysteria in all of us. But the great majority of adolescents with anxiety, hysteria, or depression are not so much the victims of catastrophe as of their own vulnerable personalities.

Behavior Syndromes

Aberrations of behavior in childhood recur in adolescence with greater intensity, frequency and diversity. There may be eating disturbances: anorexia, faddiness, overeating; abdominal disturbances: constipation, cramps, diarrhea; habit patterns: nail biting, thumb sucking, fidgetiness, tics; elimination disorders: enuresis, encopresis. Most deviations emanate from disturbed interpersonal relations at home or from innate personality disorders. Anxiety is expressed by aggression, fear, tension, antisocial symptoms, lying, stealing, truancy, sexual misbehavior, delinquency. They are acting out difficulties that may reach court involvement unless underlying personality disorders are alleviated by psychiatric intervention.

Inadequate personality is the unstable, unpredictable, uncertain youth, liable to breakdown. There is a small margin of reserve and when pinched by circumstance the immature adolescent develops neurotic reactions and uncontrolled or explosive outbursts. Shielded from inadequacy, he goes through life without overt symptoms yet reveals deficient heredity, neurotic behavior, periodic illness and poor school work. There is low physical and mental voltage with lack of resilience and plasticity, a tendency to disapprove of things, to be fearful of situations, and to show any enjoyment of anything that is normal. The feeling of inferiority and egocentricity protects him from stressful situations but the threat of dissociation of his unstable equilibrium precipitates a variety of symptoms—depression, anxiety, obsession, compulsion, hysteria—all patterns of reaction rather than mental disorders. Adolescents are rarely self-consistent for the personality organization has not yet coalesced and cannot be fitted into abnormal patterns. The fact that we can understand disturbed adolescents enables the distinction between primary symptoms alleged to be the immediate result of a disease process and secondary ones which are psychogenic reactions of the personality. On the other hand, the degree of normal psychic health is not determined by the absence of conflicts, but by the adequacy of the methods used to solve them.

Sociopathic personality presents both social and antisocial behavior. Youth acts without regard to consequences in accord with immediate desires, but the desires change frequently, so there is continuous change of goals. He is unwilling to subordinate himself to others and so becomes unscrupulous, egocentric and a scheming misfit. He not only gets himself into difficulties but embroils others with him. He never learns from experience, making the same mistakes over and over again, undeterred by punishment. He is incapable of long-term play and so floats like debris on the sea of life from pillar to post, ever submerged. Emotionalism is invariable with sudden attacks of depression in response to reverses. There is self-pity, sudden anxiety, uncontrolled rage, drug addiction. There are impulsive suicidal gestures but rarely actual suicide. He may drift into criminality and join the ranks of pathological liars, seducers, prostitutes and adventurers.

The predominant inadequacy is a feeble type of vulnerable personality with irresponsibility, lack of social conscience, lack of willpower and self-determination throughout life, adding to the growing list of life failures. The aggression pattern is actively antisocial rather than just burdensome to others. It is manifested by uncontrolled and unexplained reactions with an unemotional absence of guilt or shame which enables the prosecution of unscrupulous schemes that spell ruin to others. Physical anomalies are invariable, i.e. asthenic, underdeveloped secondary sex characteristics, vasomotor instability and cerebral dysrhythmia indicating failure in CNS integration. Treatment is ever individual. The inadequate sociopathic develops stability under firm guidance but needs to ventilate his difficulty, discharge his emotions and be subjected to a steadying influence.

Addictive personality reveals drug dependence, with neurotic and character disorders. It is a basic weakness of ego control in escaping conflictual life situations in search of drug euphoria. Emotional immaturity allows only a very low tolerance to anxiety and frustration and a tremendous need for instant gratification. The narcotic effect of certain drugs gives physiological support to the regressive tendency to reestablish the carefree passive state of nirvana. The initial stimulating effect of the drug is gradually followed by the sedative effect to help youth overcome his psychological inhibitions. He falls into a dream like one who falls into the sea. If he tries to climb out into the air as the inexperienced endeavor to do, he drowns in the addictive drugs. Put youth out of his drug illusion and you rob him of his happiness in one stroke. Humanity will never be able to dispose of artificial paradises. Most adolescents lead lives at best so monotonous that the urge to escape, the longing to transcend themselves if only for a few moments, is and always has been one of the principal appetites of the soul.

Some protean adolescents consider entry into adulthood shallow and fragmentary. They seek to improvise new approaches with drugs because of central impairment of symbolic immortality, a fundamental component of psychic life. They seek experiential transcendence in the ways of mystics through psychic experience of such great intensity that time is eliminated. Adolescent hunger for chemical means to expand consciousness is probably the larger meaning of the drug revolution. The use of drugs in itself is not wrong; it is their use as a means of evasion, as a means of escape from reality and from responsibility that is morally wrong. The most important part of adolescent life—sensations, emotions, desires and aspirations—takes in a universe of illusions which science can attenuate or destroy, but which it is powerless to enrich. Every youth sacrifices truth to his vanity, comfort and advantage. He lives not by truth but by make-believe. The notion that illusions leave him with maturation is not quite true, for early illusions are supplemented by new, equally convincing illusions.

Self-induced psychoses may be harmless but most drugs produce serious systemic consequences. Marijuana is least toxic, stimulates noradrenaline and serotonin pathways in the brain and induces mild euphoria. It enhances perceptions of sights, colors and sounds, the sense of touch, the concept of time and space. Hashish, ten times as concentrated, diminishes motivation and interest in activity. LSD enhances the activity of noradrenaline and dopamine pathways while depressing the sedative effects of serotonin. The brain becomes greatly over-aroused, creating good and bad hallucinations in some and brief wonderment at the world in others, with the force of a revelation. Incomplete concepts expelled from reality transform them into one entirely satisfying presence, maintained by repeating the dose. Then simple schizophrenia ensues with a confused personal identity. Heroin provides a feeling of escape, floating euphoria. It acts on specific neurons which become addicted to it with gradual physical and moral deterioration from progressive psychosis.

Amphetamines induce euphoria, hyperactivity, illusions. The adolescent suffers not primarily from his vices or weaknesses but from his illusions. He is haunted, not by reality, but by those images he puts in place of reality. The drug stimulates a noradrenaline pathway merging with the pleasure center of the brain above the hypothalamus. The habit becomes permanent, demanding more and more of the drug to stay stirred unto exhaustion. The past and future recede and only the present counts. As the drug begins to act on dopamine networks, persecutory delusions emerge with full-blown paranoid psychosis. Barbiturates sedate all neurons of the brain and suppress all mood controls. Habitual intake produces abrupt reactions from bursting laughter to mournful tears to outright violence. The depressed neurons tend to counter the effect by activation, hence more of the drug is taken for sedation. Once the drug is withdrawn, explosive overactivity ensues with consequent depression. Persecutory hallucinations lead to marked paranoid reactions or even to suicide.

Early detection of drug taking is difficult because the adolescent conceals his thoughts and deeds from his family. Truancy from school, loss of interest in sports, disappointing work, overt evasiveness may also be an expression of the adolescent upheaval. Similarly, at home, when the youngster's habits begin to change noticeably, the moods become unaccountably disagreeable, when he comes in late at night and has no steady girl friend, or stays out over the weekend, when he is deceptive about his friends and actions, when he loses his appetite and weight, when he looks gaunt and ghastly, the same suspicion must arise.

The presence of unusual excitability, restlessness, anxiety, hand tremors, slurred speech, sleeplessness are probably due to amphetamines. There will be dilatation of the pupils, nystagmus, tachycardia, weight loss. The appearance of unusual drowsiness, ataxia, lethargy is probably due to sedatives. The development of giggling followed by a vacant look with reddened eyes, sweating and pallor is probably due to marijuana. The discovery of pinpoint pupils, persistent scratching, watery eyes, runny nose, yawning, weight loss, neglected habitus, secretive attitude, hostility, may reveal pinpricks from heroin or opiate injections in his arms. Youth always denies taking drugs.

Delinquent personality abounds in the lower socioeconomic strata, the product of alcoholics, prostitutes, psychotics or neurotics devoid of consistent parental love. There may be love in some form but it is distorted as narcissistic, overprotective, sexual or possessive. The delinquent's interpersonal relationships are characterized by mistrust, suspicion, fear, anger, jealousy, scorn and/or disinterest towards all individuals; his self-percept, by low self-esteem, uncertainty of personal and sexual identity; and self-hatred by compensatory self-aggrandizement. He may act out his resentment for others, act out his worthless feelings and self-hatred by seeking punishment or by avoiding the usual cautions against personal injury. He may need to demonstrate his feelings of worthlessness by failing in whatever he undertakes and by getting into trouble with the law. The symptoms of personality disorder involve acting out his feelings and/or internalizing his resentments. The former includes delinquent behavior in all its variations and subdelinquent behavior such as school truancy, negativeness, disobedience, lying, cheating, and fighting, temper outbursts, crying, surliness and uncommunicativeness. The latter internalized symptoms are as serious as the overt misbehavior, immobilized by conflict of feelings, of counteraggression, self-debasement and so he remains depressed, violent, sullen, suspicious, fearful and mistrustful.

Neurotic Syndromes

All psychological problems are difficulties in youth's relationship to himself leading to anxiety, insecurity, involving pride or ego but always it has to do with awareness of the self. Neuroses are the luxury of a civilization which has developed a conceptual repertoire rich enough to permit consciousness and affluent enough to permit sufficient respite from labor and immediate threats to allow time and energy for worry about the self and the future. Neurotic ill health may reveal indeterminant symptoms or a clear-cut entity that dates back to earlier years. A phobic state may develop insidiously, curtailing adolescent life by his refusing to leave the house or partake of home life. School phobia with refusal to attend school for long periods of time requires extensive treatment for maladjustment, not for truancy. Hysterical conversion states require evaluation of the total circumstances that precipitate loss of memory, repeated swoons, paralyzed limbs. Anorexia nervosa may develop gradually in emotionally immature inhibited girls who became depressed, withdrawn, resistive to psychotherapeutic evaluation. Obsessive neurosis is initiated by compulsive rituals at puberty because of extra stress and persists with remissions unto adulthood.

Mental illness usually embodies the time-honored neuroses and psychoses. The one is a quantitative deviation in human existence while the other is a definite break in the life pattern. The neurotic has insight, the psychotic has not; the neurotic is only partly involved, the psychotic is totally distorted; the neurotic makes a fair social adjustment, the psychotic is unable to do so; the neurotic can distinguish between his subjective experiences and reality, the psychotic cannot; the neurotic perceives reality, the psychotic constructs a false environment; the neurotic maintains some life drives, the psychotic, a gross disorder of all drives; the neurotic shows an understandable reaction of the personality to psychological trauma, the psychotic has a deep-seated mental illness unrelated to personality development.

Neurotic personality arises from a common wellspring of the human condition. The dynamism of the neurosis may contribute energy to the particular personality with a great range of talent, charm, kindliness, helpfulness and gaiety. Yet, the nervous adolescent tends to have more symptoms, especially anxiety and emotionalism, than the normal and generates more of them in daily life. He is more sensitive, suggestible and self-protective. He is less self-sufficient and more dependent and thus develops symptoms on small provocation. He is less affable, more moody and more variable than the normal. Nevertheless, he may rise remarkably to a difficult situation, show great valor in dramatic occurrences, meet crises with selfless devotion, but between crises, the difficult neurotic symptomatology prevails. What is more important than the individual symptoms themselves in the problem presented by the personality as a whole, taking his life situation into account? The neurotic may appear interesting even as he is engrossed with himself, unhappy, ungrateful, malignant and never quite in touch with reality. Has there ever been an age so rife with neurotic sensibility induced by trifles? The sensitivity claimed by neurotics is matched by their egotism; they cannot abide the flaunting by others of the sufferings to which they pay an ever increasing attention in themselves.

The neurotic can be just as uncomfortable and crippled in his social, familial, academic or occupational functioning as the psychotic. He often relates his symptoms to conflicts, events and attitudes to the childhood era as psychogenic residues of a difficult home situation. Neurotic symptoms appearing immediately after a stressful event are usually benign and disappear within hours or days after the stress is relieved, but those that occur without a preceding stress may persist or fluctuate for months. At times the symptoms remit and relapse as regularly as recurrent moods. Acute anxiety attacks last for an hour or two but the neurotic propensity may last for months. The neurotic life style is so pervaded with insecurity, inadequacy and fearfulness that the periods between attacks are marked by long-term, low-level anxiety. We are all prone to the neurosis of the introvert who, with the manifold spectacle of the world spread out before him, turns away and gazes only upon the emptiness within. But let us not imagine that there is anything grand about the neurotic's unhappiness.

Psychopathic personality develops superficial relationships devoid of real feeling. He has no capacity to care for people or to make true friends. He remains inaccessible and, therefore, exasperating to others trying to help. He shows no emotional responses to everyday situations, practices deceitfulness and evasion that are pointless. He knows all the primitive emotions— fear, anger, pleasure—but is oblivious of the subtler feelings of love, joy, pity and loneliness. He may have a wide circle of acquaintances whom he uses outrageously to advance his own ends. He may even possess the charm of carrying an aura of recklessness and indifference to insults very much like the heroes in detective novels. But, he does not welcome pain and lacks courage. The diagnosis of psychopathy rests entirely on the demonstration of a diminished or absent capacity for personal relationships, rather than on the basis of antisocial activity which can occur in any mental disorder. There is a history of early neglect at home or separation from parents leading to irrational, ill-motivated behavior, stereotyped inhibition, marked self-destructive tendencies.

Depressed personality is characterized by transient attacks of the "blues" through longer lasting mood changes, to distressing dejection, rumination and hopelessness. Suicide is fifty times higher among depressed adolescents than the general population and so demands scrutiny. Three personality groups reveal depression: the first reacts to his hostile, aggressive impulses by over-seriousness, sombreness, over-conscientiousness; the second develops traits which deny hostility and utilize reaction formation by overly complaining, overly polite subservience; the third employs obsessive, compulsive habits to master these impulses leading to anxiety and agitation. Adolescent depression is masked by discord, temper tantrums, hyperactivity, running away or school failure. Youth has difficulties in handling aggressive impulses, turning them outward against others instead of inward against himself. Indeed, he attacks others to avoid the internal pain of depression, but he cannot keep up the attacks and finds himself alternating between aggression and depression. Physical disorders mask depression in the form of headache, digestive disorders, psychosomatic difficulties and accident proneness.

Cerebral excitatory pathways in the depressed gradually decrease in intensity; the mental firmament fades in illumination; the sensations are steeped in gloom. Noradrenaline and dopamine are underactive, arousal is submerged, depression emerges. Youth becomes muted with depressed thought, feeling and action, doomed outlook, overwhelmed by despair. Self-accusations preoccupy his dimming thoughts while conflicts between the ego ideal, the self-concept and body image lead to a sense of emptiness, loss of faith in people and the self, with consequent depression and maladaptation. But if these conflicts result in temporary psychic injury and improved internal demands, the process of development has gone forward. Each internal loss causes a feeling of emptiness and depression which lasts until self-esteem is restored through achievement of identification or development of a new loving relationship. Actually, depressive state in the adolescent is encouraging for it shows the ability to internalize conflicts and realign psychic forces into more mature patterns. Self-esteem, however, depleted too far leads to emotional maladaptation. The immature adolescent usually suffers from helplessness overwhelmed by the demands of the outside world in the face of depleted self-esteem. He may feel too helpless to struggle and decide that nothing is worthwhile. Or, he may see the world as untrustworthy and withdraw into fantasy. In all of these states—depression, apathy and schizoidism—there is always a feeling of hope for the future.

Obsessional personality is manifested by extreme meticulousness, undue caution and over-conscientiousness. The adolescent gets something into his head and it turns into a revolving wheel that he can't control. He weighs each pro and con with a spirit of anxiety, always making sure about everything, checking and rechecking his work, ever steeped in his routine with a place for everything and everything in its place. He shows persistent unsatisfiable ways of thinking, attempting to unscrew the inscrutable. He is ever irked by symptoms and preoccupied by his health, though his endurance is optimal. He becomes over-altruistic instead of selfish, excessively clean instead of messy, abiding instead of rebellious. His obsessions and compulsions are ritualistic, all repetitive in action, designed to prevent imaginary catastrophe. It is an escape of inner impulses in an attempt to neutralize them: a forbidden impulse is neutralized by a friendly thought; a sexual impulse by a compulsive act which makes everything seem all right. Two kinds of obsessionals are encountered—the obstinate, morose and irascible, and the vacillating, uncertain and submissive. Neither can handle money and time rationally; stingy or prodigal, or both, alternately.

Psychotic Syndromes

Adolescence as a disintegrative process seems like a psychosis itself, hence the difficulty of differentiating between normal and pathological phenomenology. In true psychosis the initial symptoms are already manifest in childhood, but the breakthrough of the psychosis needs a soil of disintegration. The content of the psychosis in childhood is characterized by simplicity and in adolescence by more varied, more complex ramifications comparable to the adult disorder. Several factors favor the development of psychosis—the time factor involves a predisposition passing through the period of latency; the age factor involves the disproportion between the adolescent's capacities and society's demands; the provocative factor involves adolescence's period of increased vulnerability; the psychopathological factor involves a profound impact on all adolescent disorders; the genetic factor involves pathologic function of a familial tendency.

Schizoid personality abounds in schizophrenics with shyness, aloofness, introversion, withdrawn behavior and autistic thinking. The brain's modulation goes out of control, as voices, visions, perceptions, delusions take over the mind. The excitatory activities of the noradrenaline and dopamine pathways are markedly increased, the conscious cortex becomes greatly aroused by excessive input. The simple schizophrenic becomes muted, withdrawn socially, develops shallow emotions and indifferent feelings about himself and everyone else. His silent mood characterizes his odd behavior, peculiar habits, nonconforming raiment. He seeks isolation in life and work as a loner with minimal personal contact—introverted, withdrawn, seclusive—living an undemanding routine. The dreamy, bearded, sandalled denizen is often a schizophrenic just as much as he is the wild-eyed adherent to some political or missionary sect. The schizoid woman becomes a cold prostitute. The schizoid process may become hebephrenic, fulminant at puberty, precipitated by stress. Everything becomes hazy, confused, bizarre due to excessive stimulation of noradrenaline and dopamine pathways. There is gradual weakening of mind and will, development of meaningless rituals, unravelling of strange hallucinations—while youth drifts aimlessly about his world.

Hysterical personality torments youth not only by ceaseless irritation with current things or by groundless anxiety about future misfortunes of his own manufacture but also with unmerited self-reproach for his own past actions. He craves to appear more than he really is, manifesting marked ability in self-deception. He pictures himself in dramatic and romantic roles but his emotions are shallow, though vivid. He is easily influenced by people or ideas, dedicated to transient ideals. The enthusiasms are sentimental rather than realistic. Confronted with difficulties, he takes flight into emotionalism rather than pursue some effective action. He is immature in his thinking, superficial in his emotions and incapable of long-term affection or sustained sexual relations. Emotional instability, vivid fantasy, and unreliability make the hysterical personality untruthful although he himself believes he is honest and frank.

The hysteric is highly egocentric in both talk and appearance, ever conspicuous about the demands he makes on people around him. There is a theatricality of behavior and a desire to impress and gain sympathy, a contrast between shallowness of feelings and intensity of their expression, and between external shyness and intense erotic interest, a lack of persistence of emotion and of effort and compensatory daydreams. Most often the hysteric is a woman, dependent on a parent, sexually frigid, prone to react with sudden spites and to dominate others with tempers, whims and suicide threats. She craves exclusive love and total attention but gives nothing in return. Many hysterics have some underlying disorder to account for the explosive symptomatology since a valid diagnosis awaits development of the syndrome.

Paranoid personality is supersensitive and rigid in interpersonal relations, ever jealous, envious, overbearing, self-important, full of grievances, suspicious of the evil motives of people. There is no real adjustment to society, with the blame placed upon others for the maladjustment. The brilliant paranoid schizophrenic emerges in a world of delusions with feelings of persecution. He is hypervigilant, suspicious of everything and everybody but philosophical about his transcendent plight. Certain characteristics encourage the development of paranoid trends. The rigid have more difficulty in adjusting than the adaptable; the aggressive are more aggrieved than the submissive; the conceited feel more slighted than the humble; the oversensitive always see significance in the casual attitude of others. Dullards are fearful and so their attitudes are exploded by apprehension. Sometimes all these characteristics are combined in varying proportions in one sensitive personality, compounding difficulties day by day, by restriction of freedom, continued frustration and prolonged failure.

Cycloid personality is the extroverted good-natured adolescent of manic-depressive families. There are three bipolar phases: (1) anxiety, (2) confusion and (3) motility psychoses. Each has an excited and an inhibited pole with any one phase of the illness unipolar or bipolar. Generally, there is emotional warmth, sympathetic responsiveness, adaptable responses, preferring activity to contemplation. But nature is never tidy and so not all who are liable to normal swings have these engaging characteristics. The one whose mood veers downward takes to alcohol; the one whose mood veers upward becomes an excited paranoid. The mood-swings from euphoria build up free energy as noradrenaline activity increases. Excessive excitement about anything and everything leads to little cerebration and no accomplishment. He talks incessantly, creates flights of fancy, flies into a flash rage. Then the manic becomes exhausted, overtaken by clouded consciousness and depression in the recurrent cycle. Mild, regularly recurring mood shifts last for weeks or months without disastrous behavior, provided youth learns to recognize his symptoms early enough to report for treatment at the first sign of trouble. It takes an enduring relationship with a physician for patient and family to collaborate.

Medical Management

Every adolescent disturbance bears an emotional component. It may not be apparent to the sufferer, but however slight, it is somewhere registered in the CNS. Troubled youth comes to the physician with turbulent feelings. We have but to listen in all honesty to hear the age-old saga of youth trying to become a man. If we listen well and with compassion, we shall find that this seemingly simple process will fill the adolescent patient with life and love and enable him to reach out like Blake's "Glad Day" to embrace maturity with the challenge, the passion, and the glory it deserves. Some personality problems can be solved by knowledge, some by experience and some by understanding, but the application of all three features yields clinical wisdom, indispensable in adolescent medicine. The complete diagnosis is the total conception of the relationship between the patient as a person, the disease as part of the patient, and the patient as part of the world in which he lives. The art and science of medicine is imbued in kindness and veracity: the wish to help and above all to understand youth in distress, the discipline to withstand all temptation to depart from scientific accuracy, and the determination to advance the adolescent cause only with the search for truth.

Adolescence represents a crucial stage in the epidemiological cycle of mental illness. Behavior is a continuous dynamic process in which the adaptive functions of one stage become the internalized structure of the next. Disturbed adolescents need outpatient programs with a broad spectrum of coordinated facilities for prevention, diagnosis, treatment and rehabilitation in schools, community and hospitals. Schools encourage the development of normal mental health, recognize mental problems early, involve troubled youth in individual or group guidance and refer problems to clinics for psychotherapy. Community agencies provide psychiatrically oriented educational programs and workshops for parents and para-professionals in cooperation with social and recreational facilities. Adolescent clinics provide individual, group and family psychotherapy and psychopharmacology. There should also be outpatient psychiatric clinics, day hospitals, group homes, emergency centers for troubled adolescents.

The care of the adolescent mind is the most noble branch of medicine. Recent advances in the electrochemistry of the brain reveal the mechanism of thought, feeling and perception, but little, if anything, on the chemistry of the brain disorders. Nevertheless, a series of remarkably related compounds called antipsychotics affect the mind and alter behavior. Their molecules mimic the shape of noradrenaline and dopamine and block enough receptor sites on neurons in the brain pathways to diminish the overactivity of these chemicals. The severely depressed respond to antidepressants that accelerate the efficacy of the arousal pathways and bring the mind up to its proper level of mood. The energy set free by the magic agencies of hope, courage, desperation, fanaticism, or by the enthusiasm for a great cause may reveal the possession of a force undreamed of, or so husband the resources of the body as to keep the flame burning long after the oil seems exhausted.

The choice of the newer chemical armamentarium depends on

criteria that help the doctor determine the meaning of the adolescent's disturbed thinking, mood and behavior. Are the disturbances simply normal variants of human experience? Are they one of the more or less clearly defined neurotic or psychotic syndromes? The neurotic builds a castle in the air; the psychotic lives in it. Are they the sequel or precursor of another disorder? Current diagnostic criteria are often insufficient for answering these questions. This is not surprising, for any heuristic effort to divide the broad spectrum of psychic difficulties into discrete entities must make artificial distinctions. To see an adolescent with any understanding involves a relationship, and into this relationship our feelings will inevitably enter. The important thing is for us to try to become aware of our feelings and when they are so intense that they cloud our judgment, we must try to face ourselves squarely and look for the trouble spots here. Medical science cannot control the mind. Surgeons can remove areas of brain, physicians can destroy or deaden it with drugs and produce unpredictable fantasies, but they cannot force it to do their bidding.

Feeling states are controlled by dual, chemically coded systems subserving pleasurable and painful reactions; the one depends on noradrenergically mediated activity in the medial forebrain bundle, the other on cholinergic mechanisms in periventricular gray region of the hypothalamus. Drugs which tend to increase the concentration of monamines at their central neuroreceptor sites elevate the mood levels. Conversely, drugs which decrease the concentration cause depression. An adolescent able to experience normal pleasurable affects but congenitally less sensitive to painful affects would be considered very stable, well adjusted. However, genetic or congenital decrease in the capacity for pleasurable affects would make him prone to depressions and readily addicted to amphetamines. In the same way, an adolescent biologically predisposed to painful sensitivity tends toward chronic anxiety with addictive reactions to alcohol or tranquilizers or to neurotic behavior.

Psychotherapeutic drugs cannot be classified in terms of brain structure or function in health or aberration. The most useful approach is based on target symptoms, disrupted patterns of behavior and/or stress factors. Minor tranquilizers are antianxiety compounds, i.e. meprobamates effective in mild neurotic-anxiety tension states. They work quickly with individual doses without waiting for cumulative action. However, they are not indicated in chronic anxiety states, schizophrenia or depression. Major tranquilizers are antipsychosis compounds, i.e. phenothiazines, effective in severe anxiety states, manic attacks, catatonic excitement and withdrawal. Maximum effects in the acute psychotic state may not be reached for six weeks, hence treatment must be continued long after symptomatic relief is obtained. Antidepressants are energizers, amphetamines stimulate the cortex, act quickly to change the mood; the iminodibenzyls overcome psychotic depressions; and the oxidase inhibitors clear neurotic depressions. We must distinguish between drug action and drug effect in the individual adolescent with a personality disorder.

Disappointments in treatment have resulted from the incorrect choice of drug, inadequate dose levels, too short treatment periods and the failure to understand drug treatment as but one phase of the comprehensive care of the patient in which the doctor-patient relationship is an integral part. The tragedy of the adolescent patient is not that he loses but that he almost wins. To him doing is overrated, and success undesirable, but the bitterness of failure even more so. He becomes a stranger in his own house. Nevertheless, failure in treatment planning is not complete in any sense. The lessons had been slowly learned by the family, changes had taken place in their attitudes, and some wholesome maturation did take place. Developmental success is never immediate, mental acuity never optimal, emotional stability never adequate. The important thing is not to overlook the inborn mechanisms for integration and maturation of the personality in due time even though it is the longest distance between two states.

Prognosis for adolescent psychiatric disorders is possible for the near future, but not for the distant future. The effects of maturation which lead to better personality integration are uncertain, while the circumstances of the youth's future environment is unknown. Some changes are helpful, initiating expanding working life, emancipation from the home, widening social horizons, developing new friends and more active sexual life. Home troubles wane, new troubles arise, but troubles persist to plague the disturbed mind. Families forgive the doctor for wrong diagnoses, but not for wrong prognoses. Adolescents with behavior or neurotic disturbances improve with time, except for the severely phobic adolescents and the marked obsessional neuroses. Insidious schizophrenia has an ominous outlook while other psychoses have an uncertain future. Prognostics do not always prove prophecies—the wise clinician makes sure of the living course of mental events. Solving the problems of disease is not the same thing as creating health for the troubled adolescent. Health and disease merge into each other, but well-being makes youth feel that now is his best time of the year. Maintaining his health and maturity demands wisdom beyond drug therapy and vision that lies beyond the complexities of youth in coping with his world.

PERSONALITY MATURATION

Man is master of the universe but not master of himself without adequate and balanced maturation. A well-developed adolescent is not merely a highly individualized individual but a highly integrated personality who crosses the threshold from childhood self-consciousness into adolescent tangled thoughts. Yet he is ready to integrate the self with the outer world and integrate all components of the self with the inner being to transform all experiences of body and mind into purposeful knowledge for further maturation. Every adolescent is in himself like a vital building. In the lower stories he lives with his animal needs, animal greeds and animal passions. Woe to him if he neglects the first, ignores the second and pretends to be free of the last. No matter how high he may rise, he must never lose sight, never cease being aware of the animal basis of his nature. If he does, he loses the sense of things, gets vapid, vague, hypocritical, arrogant, insolent. His structure turns into a tower of Babel, its builder confounding, hence doctors always wonder why so much "goes right" and parents wonder why so much "goes wrong" during the wondrous diversity of youth's private life, the only real one extant. Understanding the variations in biological growth and the concomitant sexual maturation in both sexes requires a prior knowledge of the normal range of development in body and mind. Immaturities, aberrations and afflictions then become clearer as variants of the normal rather than processes which arise without meaning or reason.

Personality Maturation Tests and Measurements

Anderson, J. B.: *The Prediction of Adjustment over Time. Personality Development in Children.* Austin, University of Texas Press, pp. 28-72, 1960.

Aronfreed, J.: The origin of self criticism. *Psychol. Rev., 71*:193, 1964.

Bennett, E. M. *et al.*: Men and women: personality patterns and contrasts. *Genet. Psychol. Monogr., 60*:101, 1959.

Bloomer, R. H.: Identification figures of boys and girls under varying degree of implied stress. *Psychol. Rep., 15*:635-642, 1964.

Buss, A. H.: *The Psychology of Aggression.* New York, Wiley, 1961.

Dick, H. R.: The measurement of morale of handicapped children. *Cerebral Palsy Rev., 25*:12-16, 1964.

Dornbusch, S. M. *et al.*: The perceiver and the perceived: their relative influence on the categories of interpersonal cognition. *J. Pers. Soc. Psychol.,* 1965.

Douvan, E. *et al.*: *Adolescent Girls.* Ann Arbor, Surv. Res. Center, University of Michigan, 1957.

Harris, D. B.: Sex differences in the life problems and interests of adolescents. *Child Dev. 30*:453, 1959.

Harrower, M. *et al.*: *Creative Variations in the Projective Techniques.* Springfield, Thomas, 1960.

Hovland, C. I. *et al.*: *Personality and Persuasibility.* New Haven, Yale University Press, 1959.

Kagan, J. *et al.*: *Birth to Maturity: A Study in Psychological Development.* New York, Wiley, 1962.

Kohn, M. L.: Social class and parental values. *Am. J. Sociol., 64*:337, 1959.

Rabin, A. I. *et al.*: Some personality characteristics and attitudes of delinquent adolescents. *J. Offender Therapy, 8*:29-36, 1964.

Sanford, R. N.: The dynamics of identification. *Psychol. Rev., 62*:106, 1955.

Santostefano, S.: An exploration of performance measures of personality. *J. Clin. Psychol., 16*:373-377, 1960.

Sargent, H. D.: *The Insight Test.* New York, Grune & Stratton, 1953.

Terman, L. M. *et al.*: *Sex and Personality* Studies in Masculinity and Femininity. New York, McGraw-Hill, 1936.

White, R. W.: Motivation reconsidered: the concept of competence. *Psychol. Rev., 66:*297, 1959.

Young, W. C. *et al.*: Hormones and sexual behavior. *Science, 143:*212, 1964.

Personality Norms

Normality as well-being is the traditional clinical designation in the absence of manifest physical aberrations and/or psychopathology. It means clearing adolescents from grossly observable signs and symptoms in order to achieve a reasonable rather than optimal state of functioning in body and mind. But each adolescent is a bearer of an iceberg with two-thirds of his difficulties concealed and only the peaks subject to examination and correction. In other words, there are always latent manifestations after the manifest disorders have been corrected or eliminated. Normality as Utopian represents an harmonious optimal blending of the diverse forces of body and mind which culminate in self-actuation. Adolescence by nature is an interruption of peaceful growth and development, hence any upholding of a steady state during this interim process is in itself abnormal. Indeed, every normal adolescent is only approximately normal, for his ego may simulate the psychotic state at any point on the scale ranging from absolute normal to absolute abnormal. Normality as average is the statistical approach based on the bell-shaped curve of probability. It represents multi-gene effects in personality characteristics that are normally distributed in the population. Consequently, an adolescent within one or two standard deviations of the mean is normal while both extremes connote retardation and genius, respectively. In applying the probability curve to adolescents, we consider the middle range the norm and both extremes the deviants in sharp contrast to the clinical and Utopian perspectives of normality. The statistical concept of normality is therefore meaningful, only when applied to average reaction time, average perceptual discrimination, average personality traits.

Every adolescent represents both a unit of personality and the individual fashioning of that unity. Youth is both the picture and the artist. He is the artist of his own personality, but as an artist, he is neither an infallible worker, nor one with complete understanding of body and soul; he is rather a weak, fallible and imperfect being. There are three layers of personality: (1) the constitutional, manifest by body build (linear, lateral or muscular); by version (extrovert, introvert or ambivalent); and by inborn intellectual capacity; (2) the developmental, manifest by psychosexual activity; oedipus complex in personality integration; and (3) by the situational, manifest by the innate ability to utilize the other two forces in order to crystallize the life style of his personality in the making to adjust his unstable environment in the interest of a fuller and happier life for all. The adolescent personality is a vital fabric that covers every facet of his internal and external adjustments to life. It is a unique pattern of self-concepts, abilities, beliefs, habits, attitudes, interests, emotions, propensities and character that distinguishes him from other individuals and displays continuity over time. Objective organization of attitudes enables him to establish and maintain relationships with other persons.

Personality is an illusion to a present state of neural organization inferred from past behaviors, expressed in terms of the probability of future behaviors. The normal personality is really an abstraction; to describe it is to describe no one. The adolescent range of normal variation for both sexes is enormous and multidimensional. The normal is a picture we fabricate of the common characteristics and to find them all in a single individual is hardly to be expected. Actually there are no adolescents, there are only personalities. None has a perfect body with perfect metabolism, and none has a perfect inner life. They are all organized with active infantile and magical processes going on within them, at the same time that they are behaving adequately as relatively mature beings. There is not the slightest possibility of eliminating all these irrational unconscious components; and if there were, they would lose all of their warmth, most of their ideals and the greater part of their feeling. They would then be nothing but automatons, with receptors, internal hook-ups and fully predictable, measurable output. But they would not be human beings. All adolescents operate at different levels of maturity and rationality; their learned adaptive ways of life and their defensive organization keep them unaware of these immature and irrational components of everyday behavior.

Adolescent maturation thus provides a fascinating spectacle with infinite variations on the theme of human metamorphosis. The component parts of the personality become integrated into viable systems despite genetic defects, constitutional disturbances, maturational patterns, developmental stages or unstable environment. All component parts of the integral systems are interdependent in such a manner that when one strays from the norm there is an automatic counteraction of the others to maintain homeostasis, whether circulatory equilibrium, electrical control, enzymatic feedback, or intrapsychic informative processes. The clinician readily recognizes without the aid of intricate tests which adolescent is developing normally at home, in school, in extracurricular activities, and in the art and science of living. He has no difficulty in noting the backward, the maladjusted, the misfit and the troubled youth. Without much formality he usually has a clear picture of the etiology of the disorder whether organic or characterological, on the one hand, or functional or situational, on the other.

Sympathetic and discerning questions yield information that enlarges the doctor's horizon of the dramatic and bizarre beyond the prosaic and the routine. Does the adolescent have a sense of well-being, good tone, vigor? Does he experience an occasional ache or pain, an occasional fit of anger or gloom yet emanates well-being? Does he resort to sublimation as the main mechanism of defense in which displaced, aim-inhibited gratification will recompense for frustrated drive fulfillment? Does he have an acceptable channel for expressing primitive urges whose more naked appearance conflicts with personal ideals or social standards? Does he learn to forego present for future pleasures to cultivate a mature ego? The immature youth wants what he wants when he wants it and cannot wait an hour to get the same thing with less trouble. Does he develop an intact sense of reality? The real world is not easy to live in; it is rough. Without the most clear-eyed adjustments youth falls and gets crushed. Reality is always material reality: hard, resistant, informed, impenetrable and unpleasant. Does he present good interpersonal relationships? Youth learns noninterference with others' peculiar ways of being happy as long as they do not interfere with his personal way of life. All relations are in no sense permanent, save in appearance, but are eternally fluid as the sea itself, yet there is no hope of joy except in human relations. Does he cultivate optimal adjustments to reality if there are no excessive social, religious, economic or occupational problems and no "drug hang-ups"? All conditioning aims at making people like their inescapable social destiny. Adapt or perish, now or never is nature's inexorable imperative.

The normal or integrated personality is adequate in structure, balanced in function, and effective in control without manifestations of local or systemic disorder. Youth bears an invisible garment woven around him from early childhood. It is made of the way he eats, the way he walks, the way he greets people, the pattern of woven tastes and colors and odors which the senses spin in childhood. He strives for a post-adolescent feeling of self-security and self-esteem without exaggeration in either direction; develops self-assertive independence of thinking and judgments; cultivates a satisfactory working capacity in the cause of his chosen vocation; enjoys a gratifying avocation and a sport or hobby; makes friends of both sexes and maintains adequate relationships with colleagues; gives and accepts love from a suitable partner to evolve a satisfactory sexual relationship with his mate; confronts himself with his own inadequacy and transgressions without excessive anxiety or reproach; withstands a fair amount of deprivation or loss; performs his excretory functions without guilt or anxiety. Adolescent equilibrium is primarily internal but exacts vast external experience for its establishment. It may be impaired or destroyed by life's vicissitudes, but compensated and reinforced by sound infantile and childhood foundations.

The clinical concept of the normal adolescent is purely relative, varying in different cultures and at different levels of economic and social integration and in different mutations with the sex and age of the adolescent. A healthy maturing personality reveals realistic self-esteem, consistent affectual relations, continued accretion of a reservoir of internal rules, a flexible sense of identity and a capacity to organize behavior relative to situational requirements. Any of these may facilitate or handicap but inner disturbances at critical periods act on the susceptible adolescent systems. The healthiest person has the largest repertoire of internalized roles so that his adaptation is effective in a wide range of transactions. The homoclite is thus limited, the borderline restricted, yet even he can adapt within a protective environment. Aberrations require delineation for diagnostic, prognostic and therapeutic purposes. An adolescent may prove to be backward or recalcitrant through no conscious desire to be difficult, as the result of mental deficiency, emotional imbalance, impaired perception, defective hearing, vision or speech. Whatever the disorder, it is analyzed in much the same manner as a disturbance in respiration or circulation and cleared or improved accordingly.

Personality Selves

Youth is an integrated machine by birth but a multiple self by experience, an embodied paradox, a bundle of contradictory selves, a history of the world for his very selves. He begins with a subjective stable self-concept of the body as distinct from the external world, develops an expressive self-concept that regulates external behavior, and finally applies his self-concept to crystallize gender-role, sex-role, identity, and self-esteem. Acceptance of his real self is the first step toward maturity. If youth grows in his psychosexual existence, he forms a creative self; if not, he becomes an authoritarian self. The self is the symbol of his own organism; the self-process, the continuous psychic recreation of that symbol. There are three selves: the self which the adolescent sees in himself; the self he believes others see in him; and the self which others really see in him.

The image of himself which he tries to create in his own mind in order that he may love himself is very different from the image which he tries to create in the minds of others in order that they may love him. There is no youth so bound to his own face that he does not cherish the hope of presenting another to the world. The ego thus presents a changing self which must be synthesized with abandoned and anticipated selves. One may understand the cosmos, but never the ego; the self is more distant than any star. Identity formation thus has a self aspect and an ego aspect. The special character of the self lies in its experience not of nature, but of others. An adolescent enters the lives of others more directly than he can enter nature, because he recognizes his own thoughts and feelings in them. He learns to make theirs his own and to find in himself a deeper self that has the features of all humanity. The knowledge of nature teaches him to act; the knowledge of self, to be; it steeps him in the predicaments of life; it makes him one with other creatures: those who serve his ambition and those who are assumed rivals.

Adolescent struggle is portrayed by Vigeland in a great column formed by the bodies of people, some trampled down, others climbing up and over the column of bodies to the summit. At the other extreme of the spectrum there are the selfless who do not participate in the game of lifemanship. They are the truly meek and the humble of the Gospel and cannot be confused with the counterfeits by the haunted expressions on their faces. Conscious experience is all that is given to youth in his task of trying to understand himself. There are two kinds of reality—the existence of consciousness and the existence of everything else. The whirl of what we call the material world has a second order of reality in contrast to the reality of conscious experience. The adolescent's inability to describe his consciousness adequately and to give a satisfactory picture of it is the great obstacle in his acquiring a rounded picture of the world. To deny the reality of the inner world is a negation of all that is immediate in existence; to minimize its significance is to depreciate the very purpose of living.

"Know thyself" is the tantalizing admonition to the adolescent. To him there is nothing of the world that seems as acceptable as his very self. But this very intimacy obstructs knowledge without exacting discipline. Self-love is a protective pride that covers his weaknesses. The self must be divested of its sense of security for the evil he commits is due to defective thinking and distorted feeling. The self never acts on rational promises, for youth's conduct is charged with ambiguities. Knowledge is not enough to achieve self-knowledge. Rational analysis of the self must not only plumb the lower depths but assess all higher ones possible. Each analysis must reveal the self from within and from without for self-direction and self-education. Self-knowledge may begin with any evaluation—Loyola's discriminating assessment of sin, Korzyski's analysis of speech habits, Freud's interpretation of dreams, Rorschach's ink blots, Murray's pictures, Alexander's postural evaluation.

The self is no fixed entity revealed in action through time. Self-inquisition enables youth to understand himself and his blind drives, overcome his negative potentialities and his unconscious distortions, and release latent potentialities which outside pressures or inner feelings have suppressed. Self-knowledge is essential for cultivating humility to neutralize excessive self-esteem and arrogant self-assertion. The adolescent is but an embryo of the self that must be brought to birth for fruition. The Socratic injunction, "Know Thyself," the Aristotelian injunction, "Realize Thyself," the Christian injunction, "Repent and Renew Thyself," the Buddhist injunction, "Renounce Thyself," and the Romanist injunction, "Perfect Thyself," are all essential steps for self-transformation into full maturity.

The inner life is a place where we live all alone and that's where you renew your springs that never dry up. Every youth hears voices that tell him that much of his current life is actually hateful to him, that many of the impulses that he has suppressed for conformity are actually those that should be obeyed. The question for the adolescent is not what he will think and feel but what he will do to achieve optimal maturation. Before his new structure can be built, he must first clear the ground, cast off his childhood apparatus, break the image, abandon glib routine, challenge the existing order, and return to his naked self with his cosmic overself. Epicurus's injunction, "Hide Thyself," is the first move towards an inner life to find one's self for a fresh start as the adolescent novice begins to face the world. Such detachment for self-examination will reveal how much of his life is cluttered with routine and how little arises out of self-need or clear conviction.

Youth dreams of daring endeavors attributing significance to more action or quick change but the more they move, the more they stand still. Discotheques and gambling, cocktails and promiscuity, drugs and dope, soporifics and aphrodisiacs, motor trips and sports are all fillers of deficient forms of life. Youth is pugnacious; he learned the habit from nature. All action veers in the direction of harm to others, for the contingencies of survival contribute aggression to the genetic endowment. Complete adaptation to environment means death, hence youth's response is the desire to control the environment.

Youth learns to hold his own in the world, not by standing on guard, but by attacking and getting well hammered himself. Violence is the rhetoric of youth even though the rest of mankind is more afraid of violence than of anything else. Youth asks a thousand questions about institutions around him but never dares ask about his true nature. Most of his energy goes into patchwork repairs and piecemeal reforms because he considers all dominant tendencies in our civilization fixed. Without a philosophy of life his goals are limited to physical security: absence of hunger, absence of disease, absence of fear, absence of war, as if by adding all these negativisms we could create a valid substitute for life. Optimal maturation requires inner autonomy. Youth must set aside fifteen minutes a day in solitude.

The adolescent must live once in the actual world and once in his own mind. Thought that does not ultimately guide action is incomplete and vice versa, action that does not in turn lead to reflection is even more incomplete. For every adolescent who is lost in abstract thought there are one hundred committed to routine action with loss of rational insight. After all, constant reflection makes life meaningful and purposeful. Life is the only art youth is required to practice without preparation, give a public performance before he acquires a novice's skill. Every youth must work out for himself the ways to modify his life in order to achieve self-direction for the fullest use of his potentialities. The intellectual needs a stiff turn at manual toil; the manual worker needs to push his mind harder than ever before. The adolescent must learn to provide for his own wants and regulate his own life without undue dependence; he must cultivate the habit of making his own bed, cleaning his own room, cooking a meal for himself or others.

The balanced adolescent treats his own situation as raw material he must mast and mold with confidence in his own powers of creation. This experience enables him to break with existing patterns and make departures on radically different lines. Such expansion and intensification of life transcends the maturing individual to high levels of accomplishment. The balanced adolescent allows a place for unpredictability; instead of being frustated by uncontrollable forces, he counts upon time to quicken the adventures of life by their very unforeseeableness. These are part of the cosmic weather whose changes enliven every activity. The mature adolescent knows bafflement, tragedy and defeat as well as fulfillment, but even in desperate situations he will be saved from despair by cultivating the consciousness that battles must be lost in the same spirit that they are won and that a courageous effort consecrates an unhappy end. With the knowledge youth acquires, he will control the power that would exterminate him; with values he creates, he can replace a routine of life based upon denial of values. Only treason to his own sense of divine can rob the new person of his creativity in the ceaseless struggle for existence.

Personality Homeostasis

Adolescent stability is but balance, and wisdom lies in masterful administration of the unforeseen. The organism has many built-in devices for maintaining a physiologically steady state or homeostasis. There are narrow limits for physical and mental changes and wide limits for psychic and social changes. Continual disturbances in homeostasis from within and without the body call into play the regulatory mechanisms to return the organism to an optimal equilibrium, ready for the next disturbance. The psychosocial homeostasis system maintains the regulatory agenda, enhanced by growth and learning during adolescence. The equilibrium-seeking cognitive structure grows larger, and more sophisticated as an adaptational system: a blow on the body is not taken passively nor will it vanish at all, except from consciousness. The body at once mobilizes its regulatory system to take care of the injury—physical, mental and/or emotional— in a determined effort to restore its original state. Even when the effect of the blow has been repaired and the organism recovers its equilibrium, the blow leaves behind a scar and a memory.

An adolescent perceives another individual not objectively but only via scanned information that is confronted with the genetic and acquired characteristics of the self. He either recognizes the other as known or rejects him as foreign. There is amazing analogy between the ways the organism scans and deals with its own and foreign protein molecules, viruses, bacteria, cells and tissues and how it scans and deals with its contacts with other beings. The behavior of the other is experienced as a gratification or a threat. Frustration induces several types of behavior disturbances which may upset the social homeostasis. When an interhuman conflict situation is not acted upon in speech or action, it persists and damages somatic homeostasis which produces psychosomatic disease. It is a form of adaptive and defensive behavior to a stress which has damaged, upset or threatened the homeostasis of the personality within its environment.

Adolescent life depends on the reconciliation of two opposite states, stability and change, security and adventure, necessity and freedom. Without regularity and continuity there would not be enough constancy in any process to recognize change. The fixed structure of determined events is the wharf on which the shuttle of free will weaves the threads of color and thickness which form the pattern and texture of everyday life. Internal stability independent of the extent of change in the outside world is the saving grace of man. But, he needs extra mechanisms to develop internal equilibria essential for survival and growth. To achieve balance without retarding growth and to promote growth without upsetting balance are the great aims of adolescent training and education. Without balance, there is deficiency in our industrial automation where borderline mentality is necessary for docile productivity in the factory with a pervasive neurosis as the final gift of the meaningless life that issues forth at the other end. Adolescent life is governed by people who know little of what lies outside and less about what takes place within it. They are unbalanced men who have made a machine out of their methods so detrimental to youth.

Youth needs stability in personality, not that of a closed system which has achieved a functional state like a crystal, but an open system constantly receiving free energy, converting it into work, dissipating it and then replenishing it over again. The dynamic balance is like that of a fountain endlessly changing, though within the pattern of change retaining it over and over again. Even the dynamic balance undergoes changes through the efforts of memory, the effects of time and events, and the new objectives of maturation. Balance in life is achieved as with walking only by a series of lunges which, in turn, are compensated by other lunges. The events that upset the balance of personality in every life further transcend far more positively than effortless ease. The hothouse fruits of life are the waxen beauty products of the best possible conditions with freedom from surface imperfections, wind and weather, worms and blights. But, fruits grown in the open have finer flavor, a richer personality and the most fascinating marks of growth and development.

The periods of highest vitality—fifth century Athens, thirteenth century Florence, sixteenth century London, nineteenth century Concord—are the peak periods in which society supported the wholeness of man. Organs and capacities and potentialities were so generally developed that every adolescent was trained to change places with any other person and still carry on his life and work. In those periods of balance, a mature, educated individual was capable of doing anything any other man could do. This view of human development contradicts the central dogma of modern civilization that specialism is here to stay. Our deepening insight into the need of the organism and personality suggests the opposite conclusion that specialization is hostile to life for it is the nonspecialized organism that is in the line of growth. Consider the ant who in 60 million years of recorded history has undergone no change. Indeed, the experience of the ant has led to no further development because of the adoption of specialization that brought perfection and stability at the ant's level and closed every route to change and betterment. The central effort in the fulfillment of adolescent life must be to bring back wholeness and balance. We must break down the segregation of function and activity within the personality and within the community.

The notion of balanced personality derives from a study of the organism internally by physiologists and externally by ecologists. A dynamic equilibrium in the internal environment is essential for well-being for minute chemical changes upset balance, impair higher functioning and produce illness. The minutiae are essential to proper functioning of the whole being to maintain balance quantitatively and qualitatively in every human activity. Balanced time is exacted by Circadian systems day and night, activity and rest, expression and inhibition. Small variations in rhythm are as important for well-being as are trace elements in the diet. Routine work which ignores rhythm and change leads to personality frustration, functional impairment and productive inefficiency. As we enlarge the sphere of interest and the field of operation we automatically increase the number of shocks and stimuli that throw the person out of balance.

We must, therefore, counteract this tendency by building protective inhibitory reactions, by lengthening the circuit of emotional responses and by slowing down the tempo of life. The world is committed to the ideology of the machine. It cultivates certain aspects of the personality long suppressed, suppresses the phases that do not fit into the mechanical world and so leads to adolescent immaturity. Every effort to overcome the distortions set up in society is devoted to the restoration of the complete human personality. Balance must be established in society before it can be fully effective in the adolescent. No amount of self-discipline can create the necessary conditions for achieving equilibrium and maturity in youth without minimizing the external pressures at work in his life. The ideal of the balanced personality must be cultivated throughout adolescence so that the physical, mental, emotional and social levels of maturation are completely integrated to function as a total unit for youth in action.

Personality Transitions

Primitives gave a face to every moving thing but modern man depersonalizes everything and everybody. Personality is considered an ephemeral property, a prison from which we must try to escape. Actually, the personal and the universal grow and fuse in the same direction. The infant has no sense of self-identity; the young child's sense of personal identity is unstable, depersonalizing himself in play and in speech; the child of five is confident of his own existence. His being in becoming is an ongoing process of growth and development. This unfinished structure bears the dynamic power of maturation until complete but never stays static. As we view adolescents year after year, the eidos of the person is realized in the personality structure with self-awareness steeped in ego function.

The control phenomenon of the adolescent spectrum is the discovery of the self as something unique, uncertain and questioning in its position in life. This search and questioning for self is the product of the adolescent's marginal role between childhood and adulthood. Deeper questioning is implied by Erikson's identity conflict with the philosophic doubting about truth, goodness and reality implied by Piaget and by Dostoevsky. A permanent state of transition is the adolescent's most noble condition. The Western evaluation is by discrete categories at each age level of the turbulent decade but the Chinese approach is that change is part of a kaleidoscopic experience contained in a continuous whole. Day and night to the Western eye are two discrete entities separated by a transitional stage, but to the Chinese they are part of one process, each being a diminution of the other. The particularism of Western thought considers adolescent development as a sequence of discrete stages, each with its own unique attributes, catalyzed into dynamic being by a delicate marriage of maturation and experience. All its manifestations coexist for clinical integration of the adolescent as a whole.

The young adolescent is becoming increasingly similar in life style to the elder youth. He loses some responsiveness to controls by adults, by the clock, the routine tasks, the dictates of conscience, the waning alliance between him and adults. Any retardation or acceleration of adolescence reaches a critical stage beyond which maldevelopment is inevitable. And damage derives equally from too little or too much, from too early or too late. Developmental injury follows incompleteness of the preadolescent stage. The libidinal and aggressive prepubescent drive is determined by the level of ego differentiation and ego autonomy during the latency period. If inadequate or incomplete, there is deficiency of cognition, memory, anticipation, tension tolerance, self-awareness, distinction between fantasy and reality, between action and thought. It is not regression because no forward development had yet been reached.

The transition into adolescence is effected when drive tensions lead to conflict formation, and resolution and mastery of the world serves as a source of self-esteem and independence. Puberal maturation precipitates instinctual tensions that make the young adolescent go backward, not forward, with oral greed, dirtiness, smuttiness, restlessness. The intensity of the regressive pull is directly proportional to the degree of independence sought. The sense of freedom from childhood dependence is ever disrupted by struggles with parents, siblings and teachers, seeking closeness and distance at the same time. The boy sets out to master the physical world; the girl, the personal relationships.

Personality structure reflects the rate of physical development. Late maturers are less physically attractive, less well-formed and more unrealistic but more sociable, more attention-seeking, more restless and immature. TAT tests showed that late maturers have negative self-concepts: feelings of inadequacy and rejection, prolonged dependence needs and rebellious attitudes towards parents. Instead, the early maturers showed a more favorable psychological picture: self-confident, independent, sociable. Children express the characteristics of age more strongly than of personality. Maturation outweighs individuality until adolescence, when introversion trends alternate with extratensive phases cyclically, w-shaped from ten to sixteen years. Around twelve years, behavior is outgoing and around thirteen years, withdrawing, followed by a reaction around fourteen years in extraversion and around fifteen years in intraversion, stabilizing around sixteen years with greater balance between intraversiveness and extraversiveness. Boys tend to be more global in approach, less productive of responses, less precise in form, producing fewer enlivened determinants. Girls give a fuller response, more detailed, more precise, richer in enlivened determinants and more responsive to human forms. Developmental changes in everyday behavior reflect growing patterns of organization of affect, intellectual approach and free energy expenditure from late childhood toward maturity according to Ames' evaluation from Rorschach responses.

Ten-year-old is easy-going, friendly, adjusted but shallow. He is intraversive, mobilizing his reserves before a new drive toward maturity gives him personalized direction. He prefers to be on the safe side, protecting himself as much as the forward thrust of development will allow like a boy on a see-saw. He protects himself positively by sticking to reality, by doing things the easy way, by identifying with the group. He protects himself negatively by restricting output, by defensiveness in inquiry, by avoiding specific detail. When his first line of protection breaks down, he withdraws in an immature way for safety. Boys act confused, girls banal.

Eleven-year-old is a paradox, lively, exuberant, talkative, aggressive, expansive. His stream of consciousness leads to confusion, criticism of the environment but not of himself, desire for adaptive inhibitions, sensitive to criticism, responsive to group pressures, creator of fantasy, formulator of precise concepts. He is highly adaptable, contrasted with superficial egocentric impulsive behavior, thoughtful reactions, independent urges combined with feelings of insecurity, aggressive yet he follows rules agreeably, is interested in others but distrustful of them. The girl is observant, empathic, adaptable, energetic.

Twelve-year-old achieves equilibrium in a new plateau of expansiveness, enthusiasm and readiness for new experience in maturation. He is a conformist willing to relinquish his dependence to assume an independent role. He has a strong sense of self. He is self-assured, assertive, and ambitious yet productive and pleasant. He is egocentric but resolves his interpersonal clashes. He is a true conformist, participates in group activity, follows rules, regulations and routines. He is sensitive about his standing with others as a realistic, practical precise being. He has feelings of incompetence and inadequacy in sex relations and turns to food as a substitute for satisfaction.

Thirteen-year-old is reflective, intraversive but blithe, mobilizing inner forces to think things through. He is charged with growth tensions that are both exciting and disturbing. He experiments with effective ways of dealing with them but exposes his immaturity. He scrutinizes, searches and worries about situations until aggressive outbursts ensue with moodiness and irascibility. He is learning to deal with new and emotional and intellectual processes for greater responsiveness to others. The girl reveals a feeble intellectual horizon in anxious obsessional, nonproductive activity that makes it difficult to adapt to the personal and social demands of everyday living.

Fourteen-year-old is self-reliant, ambitious, energetic, but insecure and inadequate, empathic. He seeks greater perspective for himself and in relations with others emotionally and intellectually. He achieves a balance between realistic and abstract concepts. He tends to be grown-up by imitation, dissatisfied with himself and his sex immaturity. He is torn between environmental stimulation and intraversive drives. The boy is interested in doing things; the girl in thinking about things. The boy is concerned with realism; the girl, with flights of fancy. The boy is outgoing; the girl prefers her own company.

Fifteen-year-old is indifferent, apathetic, withdrawn. He is sensitive, resistant and suspicious and therefore argumentative, hostile and belligerent. His responses indicate deep-seated personal and emotional conflicts as he is coping with social and religious and/or mystic and cosmic problems. It represents an integrated pattern of maturation during a period of reflective retreat, more critical for the boy than girl. He evolves his own personal and social concepts in the cause of interpersonal relationships and heterosexual adjustments to avoid being misunderstood.

Sixteen-year-old is independent, well-adjusted, well-balanced, equilibrated with himself and the world. He seeks greater perspective for himself and for his relations with others in his quest for greater self-identification and improved interpersonal relations. His objectives are not well-defined but his drive makes him pursue rewarding directions. He reveals greater intellectual and emotional expansion that leads to clashes readily overcome by the greater reserve to solve them as they occur with poise rather than explosiveness. He is ambitious, capable of defending his interests, though in search for greater self-identification and perspective. His immaturity is disguised by rationalization.

Individuality emerges progressively from the manner in which each adolescent turns all experience of body and mind into a knowledge so structured that it can be used for further growth and for action. What is more enthralling to us than this splendid boundless, colorful mutability—personality in the making. Change is the law of life but all change is not growth, as all movement is not forward. In this panorama of change naught which comes stays and naught which goes is lost. Those who look only to the past or the present are certain to miss the future. All changes in adolescent personality, even the most longed for, have their melancholy, for what youth leaves behind is a part of themselves; they must die to one life before they can enter into another. We cannot remain consistent with the world save by growing inconsistent with our past selves.

Personality Patterns

Adolescent behavior is the index of the individual; and his discourse, the index of his understanding. Behavior long attributed to an autonomous agent is now replaced by the environment in which man evolved and in which human behavior is shaped and maintained. The nomad on horseback in outer Mongolia can well replace the astronaut in outer space. Youth are like plants; the goodness and flavor of the fruit proceeds from the peculiar soil and exposition in which they grow. The background reveals the true being and their state of being. If we do not possess the background, we make the youth transparent, the thing transparent.

Adolescent behavior must be delineated to detect, measure and evaluate deviations from the normal in manifestations of man, drive for power and possession by turmoil. We must distinguish between empathic psychology and interpretative psychology. In the one, we simply try to understand the adolescent by putting oneself in his position; while in the other, we interpret what he says and does in terms of established concepts. What the physician observes of psychical manifestations is not an infinitesimal part of the psychical world distorted by pathological conditions. Just as the human physique has a long evolution behind it, the psychology of the adolescent depends upon its historical roots and can only be judged by its ethnological variants. The behavior patterns of unstable youth are universal manifestations of the final growth cycle.

Positive personality is achievement-oriented challenged by activities which require skill, not change. The skilled adolescent is realistic, although less interested in very easy or very difficult tasks, unless they are the only available opportunities. The feeling of having done something better than others is more gratifying than time-tested activities. He rarely wastes time in pursuit of the impossible nor rests content with continual mastery of familiar tasks in the face of newer realistic possibilities of accomplishment. He rarely sticks to improbable ventures when there is a more moderate risk available. He believes in greater prizes for performance of difficult feats, as an expression of pride and accomplishment and a sensitivity to the appraisal of merit. When faced with a task of considerable ambiguity, he remains confident with enthusiasm and persistence. He is ever surrounded by ambiguous possibilities and constructs for himself a world full of interesting challenge. To know youth, observe how he wins his object, rather than how he loses it; for when he fails, his pride supports him; when he succeeds, it betrays him.

Realism is not easy to live with; it is rough; it is slippery. Without the most clear-eyed adjustments youth falls and gets crushed. After all, there is no reality except the one contained within us. That's why youth lives such an unreal life. He takes the images outside him for reality and never allows the world within to assert itself. Some striking behavior reactions reveal the inner turmoil. Realism must be faced without soft concealments. The world recognizes the adolescent's ability to profit from discipline, to learn to heed warnings, to weigh consequences, to experience guilt towards those whom he has offended, to postpone pleasure in the cause of maturity. Youth must establish his own identity and find an answer to the question, "Who am I?" He must emancipate himself from his parents and obtain independence in most areas of his life. He must choose a vocation and train for success in this goal. He must cultivate the opposite sex with an ultimate choice of a life partner. He must integrate his personality towards responsible citizenship. He thus faces reality positively to achieve maturity goals or negatively to vegetate in immaturity privations.

Ambivalence reflects a disturbing interplay of discordant emotional forces. The normal adolescent is ambivalent towards persons, things and ideas throughout the final growth period. What he knows is everywhere at war with what he wants. He has the capacity to hold opposing views about most things, fights for them within himself at every turn and proves his mettle. Somehow, he can love and hate the same object or be for or against somebody at the same time and always feel the agony. The component of the ambivalent conflict is utilized to keep the other in repression.

Independence is the finest fruit of self-sufficiency. Youth wants to be independent to prove to others that he is capable of thinking, acting, feeling for himself. One way of demonstrating this ability is to attain cherished values, adult standards and community authority. But the changing patterns of his behavior from independence to dependence are ever confusing to parents. He tries his wings, reaches out into society but is pushed around by all forces and so retreats for support to his home. If his family permits him to be dependent for a while, he will regain the strength to go forth and become independent in society. Growing up is never a continuous but an advanceable pattern of development, alternating with retreats. Youth continues to function as though his helplessness had not abated, as though his security were still tied to his home, as though his everyday living depended on the maintenance of a low level of psychological tension in his significant people—resembling imprinting.

Authoritarianism has reason to fear the skeptic, for adolescent authority can rarely survive in the face of doubt. The adolescent is a master before he becomes a critic. He credits no person with good sense except the one who is of his opinion. He gets opinions as he learned to spell, by reiteration; he is determined to succeeed in whatever he undertakes; he overdoes things and appears clumsy, thus accounting for many extremes in motion and attitude. Nothing is impossible if he doesn't have to do it himself. The effective youth must know, must know what he knows, and must be able to make it abundantly clear to those about him that he knows. Youth clothes itself with rainbow and goes as brave as the zodiac.

Nonconformism is a state of mind of youth who like to stand on the margins and scoff at the babbitts. Hippies usurp the prerogatives of children—to dress up and be irresponsible. They act out a critique of the Establishment that most agree with and constitute a pilot experience of the use of leisure in an economy of abundance. The quality of the nonconformists is just as good as that of the conformists. The adolescent rebel has friends in all age groups but looks to his peer's approval for sexual identity and individual understanding. He rarely accepts counsel and guidance from adults but always turns to his age group for help. Actually, he may advise another youth as he was advised by his parents, but will not take parental advice for himself. Life cannot exist without a certain conformity to the surrounding universe and that conformity involves a certain amount of happiness in excess of pain. Indeed, as we live we are paid for living.

Negative personality has a tendency to avoid failure and thus supersedes the motive to achieve. Such youth veers toward the kind of activity in which his competence is unquestionable and shuns work requiring skill when there is any uncertainty about the outcome. He defends himself by undertaking activities in which success is virtually assured or activities which offer no chance of success because his trying to do a difficult task more than compensates for embarrassing failure. He may display dogged determination in the pursuit of an improbable goal in the face of social pressure, but will be quickly frightened away by failure at some deed that seems to him to assure success at the outset. His history of relative failure means that he will view his chances in new ventures more pessimistically than others unless there is specific information to contradict such a generalization from past experiences.

Every youth believes in his potentialities. All things are possible until they are proved impossible—and even the impossible may only be so, as of now. He is always neglecting something he can do in trying to do something he can't do. Should he fail at a task undertaken as a safe venture, he responds with a startling increase in his level of aspiration instead of persisting at the initial activity. Should he begin to sense a task rather difficult, he exhibits a marked decrease in his level of aspiration and retreats to a safer venture. These irrational moods must be understood as aspects of a defensive strategy, avoiding an intermediate degree of risk where his anxiety reaches an intolerable level. Strong anxiety is an indication of overcoming great resistance; weak anxiety, an indication that the resistance to the action is weak. The level of experienced anxiety is symptomatic of the strength of the resistance. Youth is not the sum of what he has already, but rather the sum of what he does not have, of what he can have.

Narcissism makes youth feel good and ill only in proportion to his self-love. Puberty marks the beginning of veritable unselfishness in a lifelong romance. Youth considers other people, serves the needy and develops a sense of responsibility towards self and the community. But adolescence stirs new floods of ego-centricity with a marked degree of narcissism, self-centeredness and selfishness. Some of the preoccupation reflects the psycho-physiological changes that make adolescents acutely aware of themselves in thought, feeling and appearance.

Anxiety is released from the adolescent spirit with every word and deed. As his order of existence becomes increasingly rational, its success carries with it a feeling of anxiety from the terrifying spectre of the future. Removed from his background, he is left without a function he can recognize. His growing feeling of insecurity is unmistakable and so he escapes into illness to afford protection. Adolescence is the age of anxiety, the sensed threat to the self-image. There is so much that weighs on the youth's mind and even more that grates on the nerves. Conscience and anxiety are a powerful pair of dynamos. Between them they ensure that youth shall work hard without ensuring that he shall work at anything worthwhile. Sexual feelings complicate the picture and so he is caught between the need to satisfy them and the controls set by society. Anxiety attacks by day are characterized by faintness, fear of being ill, fear of his safety or well-being of his family; actually he fears for his inability to control self-impulses, aggressiveness and hostility. Anxiety attacks by night are expressed in nightmares with falling, being pinned down, pursued or lost, symbolizing what independence will bring.

Guilt always hurries towards its complement, punishment; only there does its satisfaction lie. Adolescents who feel guilty are afraid and those who are afraid somehow feel guilty. To the onlooker, too, the fearful seem guilty. And the delusions of guilt can give rise to delusions of persecution. Youth is plagued with guilt feelings and invites punishment upon himself to obtain relief. He may seek to punish his parents by defying the law, to embarrass them in court. Insecurity develops into anxiety relieved by antisocial behavior. The next emotional response is guilt, which leads into insecurity, and then into anxiety, and then into a vicious cycle. There is a voluntary violation of the self-image that distorts all mental faculties, prevents them, confuses them. No youth harbors guilt realistically; some other be-havior reactions plague the unstable adolescent.

Fantasy is an adolescent life of internal dramas, instantaneous and sensational, played to an audience of one. Imagination is po-tentially infinite, but youth is limited to the types of experience for which he possesses organs; yet those organs are plastic, for oppor-tunity will change their scope and even their center. Youth is full of imagination and nothing that is real is alien to him. Imagination is a lake, a lofty building reared to meet the sky while fantasy is a balloon that soars at the wind's will. The adolescent's life is filled with dreaming, racing, gang fights, brutality and forms of delinquency. He needs excitement; his mind is bubbling over with rich fantasies to excite him. He must indulge in dangerous activities to release his free energy. He is not really grateful to those who make his dreams come true; they ruin his dreams. The adolescent finds it difficult to accept his finiteness, for he feels that he can do anything in the world and solve any prob-lem that he is given the opportunity to solve. There is no occupa-tion which he cannot fulfill. He indulges in wild flights of im-agination, knows no limit in fantasy and accepts grudgingly all forms of reality. But he has great difficulty in concentrating on tasks to see them through to completion.

Atheism is rather in the lip than in the heart of youth. The bigot makes the boldest atheist as a gesture of independence in challenging his parental beliefs, but he doesn't have the good-ness of heart or strength of mind to be an atheist. He becomes an apostle of practical atheism—wealth, health and power. He will leave the church, the party and the family traditions to create his own in the light of peer decisions while the abiding adolescent, on the other hand, will follow the family pattern in all realms and remain a conformist in his personal life. Religion upheavals during adolescence arise from the failure to distinguish between father and God. The two are confused, for the father is God to many children, hence a prime task is to separate father from God in the struggle for independence. It is natural for him to reject his father and so God goes with it.

Personality Perfection

The personality system of the adolescent is motivated toward action by his needs and desires in terms of goals, commitments and socialized patterns of behavior. Different needs and desires, situations and purposes elicit different roles on learned patterns of symbolic responses. The individual adolescent, however, is always more than the sum of his various roles and responses. All his acts are not only reactions but also procreations, for removal from the acts all that was possibly determined by the value of input variables will still leave something behind. This something is the personal creation of the adolescent; it is the dynamic force of procreative youth; it is the creativity for the liberation of his soul; it is youth, like Deity, that creates in his own image and unites him with the world in the process of his creation; it is youth like a tree putting forth the leaf that is created in him; and even if he loses, he will gain for a seed will only germinate if it dies; it is why human behavior is only partly predictable.

The net gain in residual personality increments increases by geometric proportions in purposes, interests and meanings from well-digested experience input, determined by innate capacity. In the final analysis, individuality emerges progressively from the manner in which each adolescent turns all experiences of the body and the mind into a knowledge so structured that it can be used for growth and for action of his whole being. Ancient youth asked, "What have we experienced?" While modern youth asks, "What can we experience?" The adolescent is what he is; he cannot be truly other than himself. He reaches perfection not by copying, much less by aiming at originality, but by constantly and steadily working out the life which is common to all, according to his innate character. Perfection consists not in doing extraordinary things, but in doing ordinary things extraordinarily well.

The adolescent is open to his experience to gauge his own feelings and activities. It is the very opposite of defensiveness, the response to experiences incongruent with the structure of the self. Every stimulus from within or without is freely relayed to the nervous system without defensive distortion. He appears comfortable with the way he behaves to fully realize his attitudes, motives and actions. He freely admits anything that he actually experiences into his conscious awareness; he behaves as if completely cognizant of what he is experiencing. He fluctuates and adapts, develops and changes continuously in the light of new experiences. His openness implies readiness to change but not to shifting his point of view with every wind that blows. His beliefs, values and attitudes are deep-seated guideposts rooted in his present and past experiences; they change because the meanings of the present are accepted and included and not because the past is ignored and excluded. The adolescent filters what he experiences through a system of learned attitudes and values; he is selective about what he admits into consciousness; he listens to some of his feelings, longings, wishes and fears, ignores or suppresses others; he tends to be authoritative, even dictatorial about his inner sensations. He realizes that it is desirable to feel, think and act in a certain way to be acceptable. His life style becomes part of his current reality for it disturbs him deeply to experience anything that will not fit. He feels freer, more whole, more in touch with the richness of his own experiences, more trusting of his own resources for meeting the demands and opportunities of life in rewarding ways as he grows into maturity.

The mature person lives in existential fashion. The self emerges from experience instead of experience being distorted to fit the self-structure. It means maximum adaptability of a flowing organization of self and personality. He is honest within himself and presents himself as he is to others; he does not need to deceive himself about his underlying feelings or desires because he is not afraid of them; he does not feel unacceptable, unlovable, unworthy or inadequate. He admits to himself anything that he actually feels; he does not need to protect himself from inner conflict, guilt or anxiety by sifting his experience; he does not need to maintain a special image of the kind of person he is at the cost of denying evidence from his own awareness. The self-concept of a congruent person is a vectorial resultant of his experiences; he adjusts his view of himself in the light of how he actually feels and acts rather than makes his conscious awareness and outward actions fit his self-concept. The real self that is discovered in his experiences truly comes from within.

The mature person trusts and depends on his own capacities to organize and interpret the data of his experiences and relies on his own judgments. He does not feel the need for external guidance, direction or authority in order to know what to do. At the same time, he is open to the thoughts others express and respects their opinions. He may use their perceptions as evidence for developing his own opinions and determining his own actions in becoming self-directed and self-motivating. He is familiar with the kind of independence that springs from rebellion against restraint; his is actually a form of dependence, for the individual is not freely self-motivating but largely governed by a persistent need to exert himself against efforts by others who would restrain, humiliate or destroy him. The mature person freely steers his own course because he knows himself, trusts his own resources and is responsible for his own actions. When results do not turn out as he expects, when he makes a mistake, he can readily see it and acknowledge it without loss of self-respect if the mistake sacrificed no principle in life. He is open to actual evidence of error or failure as well as success, and learns from experience.

The mature person reflects his basic inner qualities in all behavior. He is productive with a balanced view of his own assets and limitations based on open recognition of past encounters with people, things and ideas. He is adaptive, original and creative within the range of his potential capacity; he approaches each new situation well equipped but not committed to his past experiences. His being has the quality of a continually evolving pattern, a process with direction but with no end-point, with increasing resourcefulness in meeting both new and familiar situations of everyday life. The effective, moving, vitalizing work of the world is done between twenty-five and fifty, but the mature need to be needed, need guidance and encouragement in all endeavors.

The mature person is self-controlling; his responses are never isolated from the mainstream of experience. What he does consistently reflects a wholly unified being throughout his action. He appreciates others as he does himself; he is open with them as he is with himself, never guarded because he has nothing to conceal. He does not distrust himself to please others, nor does he use them as scapegoats for self-satisfaction. He is not afraid of liking or disliking others, of giving to others or of receiving from them, of feeling joy, anger or other emotions towards them. He expresses his feelings to others freely but not indiscriminately, for he is highly sensitive to their feelings and responds emphatically. He senses their actual feelings and meanings even when their words and notions express them only indirectly. Such mutual sensitivity draws kindred spirits to him. His empathy, congruity and openness with others, coupled with positive acceptance and appreciation that he feels towards them, help all personal and social relationships.

The mature person reveals a growing capacity to relate to contemporaries, regardless of age. It is the rebirth of a sense of fellowship with other human beings as one takes his place among them. It is the discovery of the core of strength within one who survives all hurt. It is the seriousness one had as a child on extending love to others in order to find the common denominator with one's self in divergent beings. The mature person is relatively free from the restrictive viewpoints of his self-system, able to choose his own associations and implement his own decisions, positive in the chain of cause and effect without over or underestimation of his specific role in society. Clearly, the mature individual has shed his concept of himself as a child in the adult world, has given up the particular distortions of himself and his world which he learned in his family. He has a better chance than others to attain the degree of happiness that lies in unhampered exchange of affection. He perceives pain and loneliness and experiences all empathic emotional responses—fear, anger, joy, ecstasy—with discretion.

The mature person reveals positive affirmation of his freedom from past bondage. He is free to act, assert love and be productive. This is not the pseudomasquerade of the repudiation of the needs of tenderness, which include detachment, resignation, compulsive productivity. The mature individual never commits himself unconditionally to state, church, or family, profession, or even to loved ones. If the commitment were unconditional it would cease to be the mature act, repeated affirmation of the affiliation. It would become blind obedience, the negation of one's inner freedom which is the antithesis of maturing with freedom to act on one's inner perceptions. The mature individual acquires wisdom as the vectorial resultant of education, training and experience, and a grasp of the full range of human complexity with its capacity for both virtue and vice. Such wisdom involves faith in man's ability, compassion for his frailty, capacity to sense the unknown with a high tolerance of uncertainty. The mature person grows with no foreseen limits, expands his course of satisfaction from need for intimacy, validates new experiences, and reintegrates those of the past. The mature frontiers always stay open to develop self-esteem, perceptiveness, humility.

The mature individual is a fully functioning person, dependable in being realistic, self-enhancing, socialized and appropriate in his behavior. He is a creative being whose specific formings of behavior are not easily predictable. He is ever changing, ever developing, always discovering himself and the newness in himself in each succeeding moment. Many basic personality forces, i.e. sex and eros, anger and rage, power craving from integrated to disintegrated equilibria, are deficiency needs for tension reduction, need reduction, drive reduction. The end state is homeostasis characterized by quiescence, not static equilibrium but active assimilation. Internal integration reflects a sense of unity, wholeness and oneness of body and mind and spirit in action.

REFERENCES

Allport, G. W.: Traits revisited. *Am. Psychol., 21*:1-10, 1966.
Andry, R. G.: *Delinquency and Parental Pathology.* London, Methuen, 1960.
Ayllon, T. *et al.: The Token Economy: A Motivational System for Therapy and Rehabilitation.* New York, Appleton-Century-Crofts, 1968.

Balser, B. H. (Ed.): *Psychotherapy of the Adolescent.* New York, International Universities Press, 1957.

Barnard, J. W. *et al.*: Teachers' ratings of student personality traits as they relate to I. Q. and social desirability. *J. Educ. Psychol.,* 59:128-32, 1968.

Bellak, L.: Personality structure in a changing world. *Arch. Gen. Psychiatry,* 58:91, 1961.

Bernardi, S. *et al.*: Adolescents in psychiatric care. *Br. Med. J.,* 2:3-4, 1971.

Bleuler, M.: Endocrinological psychiatry and psychology. *Henry Ford Hosp. Med. J.,* 15:309-17, 1967.

Blinder, M. G.: The hysterical personality. *Psychiatry,* 29:227-35, 1966.

Blos, P.: Character formation in adolescence. *Psychoanal. Study Child,* 23: 245-63, 1968.

Brim, O. G. Jr.: Adolescent personality as self-other systems. *J. Marr. Fam.,* 27:156-162, 1965.

Cameron, N.: *Personality Development and Psychopathology.* Boston, Houghton Mifflin, 1963.

Cammer, L.: Personality: a biologic system. *Cond. Reflex,* 6:52-61, 1971.

Carson, R. C.: *Interaction Concepts of Personality.* Chicago, Aldine, 1969.

Cattell, R. B.: *The Scientific Analysis of Personality.* Chicago, Aldine, 1965.

Child, D.: Personality and social status. *Br. J. Soc. Clin. Psychol.,* 5:196-9, 1966.

Crown, S.: *Essential Principles of Psychiatry.* London, Pitman, 1970.

Davis, J. M.: Efficacy of tranquilizing and antidepressant drugs. *Arch. Gen. Psychiatry,* 13:552, 1965.

Erikson, E. H.: Growth and crises of the healthy personality. *Psychol. Issues,* 1:50-100, 1959.

Eveloff, H. H.: Psychopharmacologic agents in child psychiatry. *Arch. Gen. Psychiatry,* 14:472, 1966.

Farley, F. H.: Comparability of the MPI and EPI on normal subjects. *Br. J. Soc. Clin. Psychol.,* 9:74-6, 1970.

Ferreira, A. J.: Loneliness and psychopathology. *Am. J. Psychoanal.,* 22:201-207, 1962.

Fish, B.: Drug use in psychiatric disorders of children. *Am. J. Psychiatry,* 124:31, 1968.

Fowler, R. E. Jr. *et al.*: A computer program for personality analysis. *Behav. Sci.,* 13:413-6, 1968.

Glasner, S.: Aberrant dependency. *Psychiatr. Q.,* 41:71-9, 1967.

Grey, J. A.: The physiological basis of personality. *Adv. Sci.,* 24:293-305, 1968.

Hall, C. S. *et al.*: *Theories of Personality.* New York, Wiley, 1970.

Hallworth, H. J.: Dimensions of personality and meaning. *Bri. J. Soc. Clin. Psychol.,* 4:161-8, 1965.

Hardwood, A. C.: *Recovery of Man in Childhood*. London, Hodder and Stoughton, 1958.

Hekimian, L. J. *et al.*: Characteristics of drug abusers admitted to a psychiatric hospital. *J.A.M.A., 205:*125-130, 1968.

Henderson, A. S.: The physiological maturity of adolescent psychiatric patients, juvenile delinquents and normal teenagers. *Br. J. Psychiatry, 115:* 895-905, 1969.

Hirsch, A.: *The Troubled Adolescent as He Emerges on Psychological Tests*. New York, International Universities Press, 1970.

Hjelle, L. A.: Accuracy of personality and social judgments as functions of familiarity. *Psychol. Rep., 22:*311-9, 1968.

Howells, J. G. (Ed.): *Modern Perspectives in Child Psychiatry*. London, Oliver & Boyd, 1971.

Judd, L. L.: The normal psychological development of the American adolescent. *Calif. Med., 107:*465-70, 1967.

Kahn, J. H.: *Human Growth and the Development of Personality*. London, Pergamon Press, 1965.

Keniston, K.: The psychiatrist and youth: joint efforts toward innovative solutions. *Am. J. Psychiatry, 126:*12, 1768, 1970.

Kernberg, P. F.: The problem of organicity in the child. *J. Child Psychiatry, 8:*517, 1969; A psychoanalytic classification of character pathology. *J. Am. Psychoanal. Assoc., 18:*800-22, 1970.

Knobal, M.: On psychotherapy of adolescence. *Acta Paedopsychiatr., 33:* 168-75, 1966.

Kraft, I. A.: The use of psychoactive drugs in the outpatient treatment of psychiatric disorders of childhood. *Am. J. Psychiatry, 124:*1401, 1968.

Kutter, M.: The influence of organic and emotional factors on the origins, nature and outcome of childhood psychosis. *Dev. Med. Child Neurol., 7:*518, 1965.

Kysar, E., *et al.*: Range of psychological functioning in normal late adolescents. *Arch. Gen. Psychiatry*, Vol. 21, 1969.

Lambert, W. E. *et al.*: Judging personality through speech. *J. Commun., 16:* 305-21, 1966.

Laughlin, H. P.: *The Ego and Its Defenses*. New York, Appleton-Century-Crofts, 1970.

Leary, T.: *Interpersonal Diagnosis of Personality*. New York, Ronald, 1957.

Lidz, T.: *The Person*. New York, Basic Books, 1968.

Lorand, S.: Adolescent depression. *Int. J. Psychoanal., 45:*53-60, 1967.

Lourie, R. S.: Adolescence: normal psychological development and psychiatric problems. *J. Periodontol., 42:*525, 1971.

Mason, R. E.: Self-ratings of personality development. *Psychol. Rep., 19:* 1179-82, 1966.

Masterson, J. F. Jr.: The psychiatric significance of adolescent turmoil. *Am. J. Psychiatry, 124*(11):1549-1553, 1968.

Moore, T. W.: Studying the growth of personality. *Vita Humana,* 2:65-87, 1959.

Norton, H. W.: Blood groups and personality traits. *Am. J. Hum. Genet.,* 23:225, 1971.

Ojha, A. B. *et al.:* The use of the Maudsley personality inventory on university students. *Br. J. Psychiatry, 112:*543-8, 1966.

Paivio, A.: Personality and audience influence. *Progr. Exp. Pers. Res.,* 2:127-73, 1965.

Peck, R. F. *et al.: The Psychology of Character Development.* New York, Wiley, 1960.

Philip, A. E. *et al.:* The reliability and utility of a clinical rating of personality. *Br. J. Med. Psychol., 44:*85-9, 1971.

Poinsard, P. J.: Psychiatric problems of adolescence. *Ann. N. Y. Acad. Sci., 142:*820-2, 1967.

Rado, S.: *Adaptational Psychodynamics: Motivation and Control.* New York, Science House, 1969.

Ramsey, R. W.: Personality and speech. *J. Pers. Soc. Psychol., 4:*116-8, 1966.

Richman, N.: The origin of personality. *Dev. Med. Child Neurol., 13:*102-5, 1971.

Roback, H. B.: Human figure drawings: for personality assessment. *Psychol. Bull., 70:*1-19, 1968.

Sanderson, A.: The relation between facial appearance and personality. *Dev. Med. Child Neurol., 12:*807-9, 1970.

Savage, P. P. E.: Psychopathology of the adolescent. *N. Z. Med. J., 68:*295, 1968.

Sciortino, R.: Personality characteristics inventory. *Psychol. Rep., 27:*612-22, 1970.

Thomas, A. *et al.:* The origin of personality. *Sci. Am., 223:*102-109, 1970.

Vinoda, K. S.: Personality characteristics of attempted suicides. *Br. J. Psychiatry, 112:*1143-50, 1966.

Walter, W. C.: Physiological correlates of personality. *Biol. Psychiatry, 3:* 59-69, 1971.

Weiner, I. B.: Psychological disturbance in adolescence. New York, Wiley, 1970.

Wiggins, J. S.: Personality structure. *Ann. Rev. Psychol., 19:*93-350, 1968.

Wolberg, L. R.: *et al.: The Dynamics of Personality.* New York, Grune & Stratton, 1970.

Zubin, Joseph *et al.: The Psychopathology of Adolescence.* New York, Grune & Stratton, 1970.

CHAPTER VIII

EPILOGUE
ADOLESCENCE 2000

If we take adolescents as they are, we make them worse,
If we treat them as if they are what they ought to be,
We help them to become what they are capable of becoming.

Adolescent life will ever be forward motion toward newer knowledge. It is the most tangled conglomeration inflamed with passion in quest of productive maturity. Molecular unwinding of the biological clock creates this self-realization of all the potentialities of atomic electron states. Much of the free energy released will be devoted to improving the eventual quality of life so that it may be joyous or noble or creative. Youth will be taller, stronger, more efficient in physical performance. His physiological metabolism will utilize the raw materials of nature more effectively in transforming them into bio-physico-chemical compounds for everyday living. His psychometabolism will utilize the raw materials of experience more effectively into psychosocial thought and feeling for more meaningful living. His homeostatic feedback mechanisms will be more efficient in regulating body tissues. His micro-miniaturized brain will be more masterful of world reality.

Youth will live as he thinks, not think as he lives. He will cease to be other people; no longer will his thoughts be someone else's opinions, his life a mimicry, his passions a quotation. He will only become better when he is made to see what he's like. His indiscriminating, illicit, incessant orgasms, devoid of romance or spirit, will replace the Cross as the focus of longing and image fulfillment. He will live violently, admired for his instinctive animal courage, but will not endure the days of his youth. He will need a faith, a hope and a purpose to live by and to give meaning to his existence. He will avoid excessive suffering and will capture the joys within his reach. He will yearn for love and relatedness to other persons. He will want to gain and to

287

hold his self-respect and the admiration of others, and he will forgo pleasures and accept pain for this respect.

The forces shaping the future phenomena are apparent, the events are in train, but the progress means war with society. Youth's desire to understand the world and his desire to reform it are the two great engines of progress, without which society would stand still or retrogress. The shape of the world at 2000 and youth's place in it will depend on the manner in which man confronts the major challenges. Social organizations, through their political leaders, will determine peace or war, conventional or nuclear weapons, growth or deceleration of populations, natural or artificial food production, conservation or degradation of a healthy environment, alignment or alienation of youth, adequate or impoverished living standards, maintenance or rejection of traditional values, uniform or disrupted monetary systems—all components of a single world problematique.

The dramatic balance between the will of the people and government will always prevent its degeneration into tyranny even though man is about the same with despotism as with freedom. We will need supermen to rule us—the job is so vast and the need for wise judgment so urgent that youth will rise or fall with the coming events. But alas, there are no supermen. We should set about planning a fulfillment society rather than a welfare society. Greater fulfillment will come about by the realization of more of human potentialities. Once youth grasps what a small fraction (about 10%) of their potentialities are actually being realized, and what vast new possibilities are awaiting to be elicited, they will have a new and powerful motive to activate their future. The task is not to foresee but to enable youth's uncertain voyage. More and more of what happens in the world is subject to human intervention and control, so that we will have the power to determine the future, rather than to prophesy it.

Adolescent Advances

"For him that is joined to all the living, there is hope." For this is the age when youth—defective, deviated, disordered—or just immature will be brought to fruition, maturation, self-fulfillment in body, mind and soul by continuing biomedical discoveries. Growth and development, potentialities and maturations, youth and age, male and female, love and hate, good and evil, health and disease will have new meanings for new possibilities. All beings will be literally more beloved for the imperfections which have been divinely appointed, that the law of human life may be effort and the law of human judgment mercy. The indefatigable pursuit of an unattainable perfection alone will give new meaning to life. The human habit of looking for perfection in everything will make all notice the shortcomings, for their sense, hungry for complete satisfaction, will miss the perfection it demands. Yet all mankind is born for perfection and each shall attain it if he will but follow the creative leaps of biomedical progress.

The adolescent body carries, in itself, a hitherto undefined principle for perfecting itself. It will unravel with the physical principles to be discovered with the aid of quantum mechanics. It may well be that life itself owes its very origin to this principle. On descending into the world of the smallest particles, the electrons and quanta, molecules enter into entirely new relations revealed only by solid state physics. Atoms are formed by atomic nuclei and surrounded by electronic clouds which may fuse over long distances, according to the laws of wave mechanics. The living state is even more complex for it not only has to improve itself but has to communicate the improved blueprint to the DNA of sperm and egg cells. The perfected living system can now adapt to its surroundings and change with it from some feedback of the periphery to the genetic material.

Biological characteristics, profoundly affected by early environmental influences, will be gradually modified in childhood. They are more than conditioned behavior patterns; they are lasting imprints in growth rate, sexual maturity, mental ability, adult size, efficiency of food utilization, and in resistance to malnutrition, to infection, to stress. With knowledge of the mechanisms through which early influences exert such lasting effects at critical periods of vulnerability, it will be possible to predict potential deviations and institute preventive measures at every stage of development to improve the course of maturation.

Social maturation will be controlled throughout childhood to subordinate impulses and interests in the furtherance of harmonious group life. Everything will intercept youth from itself. The simple truth is that to live is to feel oneself lost; once youth accepts it, he has already begun to find himself, to be on firm ground. Indeed, the adolescent who regards his own life and that of his peers as meaningless is almost disqualified for life. Psychosocial stimulation in an enriched environment accelerates brain development while social isolation reduces the cells in the cortex, cerebellum and limbic systems of the brain. Subcortical structures are affected in early life with resulting effect on behavior, while cortical structures are affected in later years with resulting impairment in intelligence.

Family caliber reflects society's status. If well ordered and well instructed they are the springs from which go forth the streams of national greatness, of civil order and public happiness. But the family cult as a nuclear unit in society will give way to group-oriented communes. Youth will develop completely antagonistic codes of behavior. As members of the group they will not only take life easily but will give up life easily. All individual reflexes serve to preserve their lives, but most of them will be ready for principles evolved by the group. As individuals, they will try to enrich themselves, but for the group they will readily give up their belongings. Human nature will remain relatively constant while human culture will become more variable. The rising generation in this country composing about 7 percent of the whole human race will hold about 50 percent of the power. The rate of change in man's environment will gather speed while youth's capacity to adapt to social change will remain limited. Intellect moves faster than emotion, hence the time lag between thought and feeling and between knowledge and response.

Youth's mind will be directed by psychotechnology to canalize development so as to reconcile conflicting drives and impulses in order to effect psychological bonds with other beings and with nature. This will correct various unfortunate tendencies to find scapegoats for his own guilt, the tendency to put off his own responsibilities on to someone or something else. It will help to prevent the discharge of aggressive impulses and hates in wrong and dangerous ways and help him to avoid reification—erecting abstractions to the states of real entities, thinking that there is any such thing as truth or virtue.

The intellectual climates will become fewer in number and poorer in quality. Knowledge of a superficial kind and limited application will be highly popular. The social and economic standing of intellectual activity will be low. The professor of theology will not know his Bible; he will write technical articles on little points of controversy at the moment, but the Bible will not flow through him to exalt his spiritual life. He will not be the vehicle for anything great; he will be a prairie in the quicksand, an agent in an anonymous moral migration that cannot write its Classic. Maintenance of high academic standards will not be easy in times of dilution of mind and money.

Active work will save youth from himself; indolence will make him a prey to useless regrets and dangerous avenues, for the soul's joy lies in doing. But work will expand to fill the time available for its completion. The cybercultural revolution will rescue youth from drudgery of work and provide him with greater opportunities for suitable education and personal enjoyment. There will be greater sensible leisure to cultivate inner resources. The ethos of hard work will wane with greater productive automation and widespread affluence and reaction to the materialism of technology, so that new life styles will evolve with a return to creative hobbies. Youth will have access to prerogatives monopolized by a few and will find fulfillment beyond material abundance.

Increased leisure and increased means will become the two civilizers of youth. To be able to fill leisure intelligently will be the last product of civilization. Will youth have the resources with which to cope with this *embarras* of temporal richness? The answer will appear to be positive for higher intellectual levels and negative for all other levels. In the past, the unskilled laborer toiled hardest and longest; in the future, it will be the intellectually gifted who will work most intensely and with deepest satisfaction. Affluence and leisure will promote aggressive antisocial behavior, sexual promiscuity, alcoholism and depressive disorders as will degraded poverty and economic exploitation. Education will settle these difficult social problems with development of talents, skills and interests with which to fill the long leisure that will become the human heritage.

Adolescent sexuality will achieve functional satisfaction without tension and clear the wind for attention, learning and creativity. The sex instinct is a prime mover of all we do and are and dream, individually and collectively, hence the coming cultivation of the degree and kind of sexuality that will reach up to the ultimate pinnacle of the human spirit in men and women. Youth will achieve emotional homeostasis, not by the measure of emotions, as religious ascetics have attempted, but by their integration, as the nervous system integrates the activities of antagonistic muscles. Understanding and intellectualizing their sensual pleasures will convert them into servants rather than masters. Negative eugenics will be possible with better understanding of its genetic basis. There will be no need to forbid marriage; few will wish to marry a spouse with whom they share a recessive gene for microcephaly, congenital deafness, cystic fibrosis of the pancreas, to transmit to a quarter of their children.

Spiritual youth will envisage himself as a convergence in the Omega: "I am the Alpha and the Omega, the first and the last, the beginning and the end." Organized religion will be abandoned by militant youth. The coming ethical view will be founded upon a moral pragmatism stressing the importance of good human relationships in all walks of life and in all social situations regardless of abstract ideas of right and wrong. How people treat one another will be more significant than what they believe. Youth leaders will be identified with the perplexing problem of oppressed communities, while youth will be on the move to help shape its own destiny. Nevertheless, many adolescents will arrive at some system of religion concerning the meaning and conduct of their lives. The view according to the temper of the mind which it inhabits will be a passion, a persuasion, an excuse, a refuge; never a check. There will be only one religion, though there will be a hundred versions of it. Adolescent life will remain a flash of occasional enjoyments lighting up a mass of pain and misery, a bagatelle of transient experience. And yet religion will come closer than work-a-day opinion to the heart of all things.

Time's arrow points toward a better future for youth based on acquired expectations. His paths toward this or that future, conditioned by constitution, temperament and talent will be largely determined by his conceptual mapping. The progressive individual will embrace changes in life styles, switch careers and social roles. The capacities of youth will be evaluated for suitable occupations without trial-and-error methods. Happiness will be doing a job which is difficult, but just not too difficult for the adolescent to drown his sorrows in complete absorption. Young men and women regarded primarily as producers will have a happier life than those regarded as consumers. The success or failure of the service-oriented society will depend on the choice of adolescents for the jobs and jobs for the adolescents.

Intelligent youth lives in the future. His well-being is always ahead. Such a pensive creature is probably immortal. He lives under the shadow of an event that has not come to pass. Apparently, the future centers into him to transform itself in him long before it happens. Youth's task is not to foresee but to enable the future; without some goal and some effort to reach it, no adolescent can live. Once he has mastered his field of endeavor, he becomes a skeptic concerning it, consequently a revolutionist. He will be content with nothing he possesses and will always be looking for something new. Youth will continue to remain strong by opposing nature or the external world as a projection of his personality, reflected by its capacity, need and culture.

Medical Advances

Adolescent practice reveals a striking shift from the physical and biological to the behavioral and social disorders because of the unique environment being created by man rather than by nature. Health and happiness or disease and disability derive not only from the physical constitution but from the social world. It takes a multiplicity of direct human contacts for the normal development of mind, body and soul throughout life. Even the most efficient methods of communication cannot replace direct encounters as the basis for a healthy, happy and creative existence. Adolescents, in particular, learn chiefly from others and most effectively as a result of I-thou relationships to satisfy the essential psychosocial requirements of maturation. Their growth is seen in the successive choice of friends since the path of social advancement is strewn with broken friendships. Young people are quick enough in perceiving and weighing what they suffer from others, but mind not what others suffer from them. They prosper only by evolving what is inherent within them and by modifying aspects of their whole being if physicobehavioral disorders thwart the gradual stages of maturation at every developmental level. The best adolescent tries to perfect himself, and the happiest feels that he is perfecting himself.

The clinical era of passive observation of unfolding events is giving way to the scientific era of active intervention in developmental episodes. It unravels defect, deviations and even disasters in the multifaceted panorama of maturation as a basis for planned modification of the constitutional makeup, home setting and environmental challenges. It is a fluid process of homonization, the final transformation of all inborn potentialities into an integrated personality. The end-product requires balanced developmental levels of the physical, mental, emotional and social at the same plateau to displace immaturity. Indeed, we are children so long, we never get over it! Clinical preoccupation with the future not only prevents us from seeing the present as it is but prompts us to rearrange the past. Life is an irreversible process, hence its future can never be a repetition of the past.

Clinical judgment is only the extent of the mind's illumination based on training, experience and wisdom. The clinician is complex—one part of him uses himself as a sensitive clinical instrument functioning through hunches, intuition, preconcepts, subjective impressions to be in communion with the relevant reality of his patient; the other side of him hankers after the stable, measurable and scientifically objective which loses meaningfulness and validity. But when working with the adolescent, he is single minded, pragmatic and utilitarian. The physician's function is to cure sometimes, to relieve often and to comfort always. Science will greatly increase the proportion of patients whose illnesses can be cured or relieved, but the decline in religious belief has greatly increased the need for comfort. The philosophic physician will therefore combine the roles of scientist and priest.

The coming cybernetic system of impersonal medicine will preclude any probability of the personal entente between patient and doctor but not between patient and computer that never wastes a word, a drop of ink, or a drop of blood. The computer will give accurate weight to all the relevant information and express the judgment in terms of quantitative probability. But there will be a long process of technical development before the machine can do more than touch the fringe of medicine. It will be displayed as a pattern or an oscilloscope rather than a definite diagnosis or treatment. The physician will interpret the pattern with the knowledge that all measurable data have been given due weight. Medical routine will be done by paramedical technicians in the health team. Rehabilitation for the disadvantaged and deprived will absorb social services while the impersonal physician will become the human biologist to every segment of society evaluating computer data and treating patients through health technicians.

Epidemic disease control will abolish infectious disease, except the common cold and other viral diseases. The forces of selection for genes acting on human beings will change drastically in the development of immunity and the fitness which diminished in the absence of disease will be gradually regained. Youth will be relatively free from nutritional deficiency diseases. Communes will still be infested with lice, the tropics with plasmodia, the underprivileged homes with venereal disease. The proposed drive to make people aseptic in order to decrease cancer by providing vitamins for intestinal function will deprive the body of defenses against sporadic infections. The untreated will be offensive and so create emotional tensions and sexual barriers.

Retarded growth will be corrected not only by the pituitary growth hormone but by its synthetic analogue and purified growth hormone from animals. It will accelerate the growth in height of emotionally deprived children whose growth retardation is the consequence of suppressed pituitary GH function. Its administration will raise the amino acid levels in blood and muscle cells throughout adolescence. Girls' muscle cells increase in number at a constant rate with muscle size attained at eleven while boys' muscle cells increase in size beyond eleven and their cell numbers increase exponentially during adolescence.

Protein starvation will be the principal cause of illness and death on the global scale in the face of excessive population for collective comfort. Of course, protein deprivation will not appear in vital statistics as immediate causes—only nonspecific infections, malaria, tuberculosis and cancer of the liver. But malnutrition will be as convincingly the prime cause of death as overcrowding, poverty and lack of hygiene were incriminated during the Western industrial revolutions.

Obesity will be prevented and controlled in terms of the increased number of fat cells in early childhood or the increased size of fat cells in later childhood. The former arises from excessive caloric intake which increases growth hormone secretion while the latter, from excessive protein intake. Whatever the cell response to the nutritional pattern, it predisposes to chronic diseases, i.e. hypertension, diabetes, renal disease. The obese suffer not so much gluttony as starvation brought on by boredom and disappointment. Nutritional therapy for weight control will be more effective supplemented by sufficient exercises for greater physical fitness of youth.

Chronic diseases, especially heart disease and cancer, will be more preventable and much more treatable by biomedical technology. Injuries will continue to plague a faster moving, faster living technologic society. Surgery will be dominated by the replacement of diseased or damaged tissues. Organic transplantation will be standard procedure. Corneal grafting will enable the blind to see again. Homologous grafts of blood vessels from cadavers will not survive in the original form but provide a framework for the permanent structure resulting from invasion by the hosts' cells. Transplantation or replacement of the heart, liver and lungs will be effective but that of the brain appears out of the question. Transplantation of organs will be commonplace once tissue incompatibilities will be overcome. Higher apes may be raised to supply suitable spare parts. Artificial contrivances will supplant organ transplantation with the development of plastic prostheses of heart or kidney.

Genetic disease will be controlled by predicting the outcome of certain human conjugations. Chromosomal and genetic abnormalities will determine the underlying basis of disease processes and thus enable correction of genetic errors at the cellular level. This will require manipulation of ribonucleic acid extracts to wrest from nature the control of inherited traits. The proposition for marriage will not be so much a matter of putting cards on the table, as between interested parties, but of putting cards into a machine to determine whether society will permit them to reproduce.

Eugenic engineering will operate at the level of existing genes to decrease the prevalence and expression of undesirable genes. These efforts will be effective in proportion to the numbers of detrimental genes which will be identified, to the development of effective methods for their detection in the hidden carrier state, and to the acceptance by individuals of their social responsibility not to perpetuate these genes. Euphonic engineering will continue to operate at the level of gene expression on the phenotype of the individual. It will prevent harmful accumulation of toxic materials associated with genetic defects by dietary restriction. Striking examples are phenylalanine in PKU, galactose in galactosemia, branched amino acids in maple sugar urine disease, isovaline acidemia involved in mental retardation. Harmful dominant genes will be repressed and inactive genes depressed, even *in utero*.

Genetic engineering will alter existing genes by direct mutation and by replacement. It will be done with liver cells grown in culture. The desired new gene will be introduced by direct mutation from normal cells of another donor by transduction or by direct DNA transfer. The rare cell with the desired change will then be selected, grown into a mass culture and reimplanted in the patient's liver. Eventually there will be synthesis of the desired gene according to the specifications of the genetic code and of the enzyme it determines by *in vitro* enzymatic replication of this DNA. Scientific treatment of a child with a genetic, metabolic, or immunological anomaly which is potentially lethal will always be extravagantly expensive. It will require a full-time team of biochemists and technicians and will subject the child to constant examinations, blood tests and injections throughout life.

Selective breeding for desirable traits will be possible for man as for animals. Mankind became extensively polymorphic in the past and retains this polymorphism at present despite genetic diversity, but gross interference with natural conditions is clearly possible. It would not take many generations to breed average Japanese of six feet or Caucasians of four feet. We could breed for leanness or obesity, wavy or wiry hair, blue or black eyes, high or low mentality, spatial perception, verbal capacity, cooperative or disruptive behavior, for selection could be effective even with traits of low hereditability. Man is potentially able to select his own genetic constitution. All-out-self-selection will be overcome by insemination of deep-freeze stored sperm of distinguished men in cases of infertility of the husband. Homo sapiens, the creation of nature, will transcend her.

Youth will relieve God of the responsibility of creation, for life will eventually be created in the laboratory and living things will be shaped, molded and modified at will. Genetically, inherited diseases will be prevented by modifying the chemical properties of the genes themselves. Each individual is chemically and biologically different from every other individual, hence the erroneous legal myth that "all men are created equal" will alter social philosophy to advance the being more realistically by encouraging individual fulfillment in accordance with the beatnik contention.

Over-population of the world to 6,000 million is in prospect by the turn of the century. In this explosion, delicately poised balances of populations will be disturbed while numbers will increase at a measured pace in affluent western-style countries. The more thickly populated will become intolerably situated, especially in multiracial cities, with the sharpening of physical and political hungers. The mechanism will create conditions favorable for the survival of the unfit and the elimination of the fit. But the rabbit-like unplanned breeding of man will give way to the God-like planned breeding exercised for domesticated plants and animals to thwart atrophy of the best qualities in man in the standing-room environment. Rational individual and social control over reproduction will be government privileged by social scientists. Human sterilization will become mandatory with scientific concern over the quality of the procreation. There will be selection for mental, physical and emotional fitness. We will have hyper-quality rather than higher-quantity progeny.

Community Advances

Science for society's sake will be the great objective of 25 million scientists by 2000 with a tenfold productivity in life sciences. The search for truth per se will be augmented for better or worse by a search for what is both morally right and attainable. The purists' motto of science for science's sake will carry less weight than the pragmatist's science for society's sake. The relative decay of fatalism will complete itself while the scientific community's new sense of social responsibility will come to full fruition. A true symbiosis between man and machine will enhance man's intelligence through collaboration with a computer, its role rising to that of a quasi-colleague. The community will be cybernated to extend youth's ability to produce in greater volume with less physical effort or mental strain. He will be joined to all the living through the machine, isolating one of our essential attributes—our kinship with nature. He will become a kind of cosmic outlaw, having neither the completeness and integrity of the animal nor the birthright of a true humanity.

Man will be living in a global village with an automated civilization of economic functionalism without a characteristic poetry, without a typical dream, without coherent painting, without aesthetic architecture. One of the great impulses of mankind is to arrive at something higher than a natural state. Art, poetry, drama, music, dance, philosophy, myth, religion are as essential to youth as his daily bread. Man's true life consists not in his work activities that sustain him but in the symbolic activities that transcend him. Then he lives a life tuned in the great intangible vistas of beauty, truth and goodness that are the heritage of civilized man.

Cultural evolution from the turn of the century will increase the complexity of the world as a superimposition of a thousand million individual patterns, the one upon the other; the rapidity of communication 20 million times, the rate of travel 200 times, the speed of computer operations 2 million times, the utilizability of our energy resources 2,000 times, disease control 200 times. This will create enormous problems of adaptation for which new sciences will emerge to cope with those adjustment difficulties. The greatest assassin of life is haste, the desire to reach things before the right time which means overreaching them. Youth in haste cannot think, cannot grow, nor even decay, ever preserved in a perpetual puerility. However, there are no conditions to which youth cannot become accustomed, especially if he sees that all those around him live in the same way.

Mankind will become so much one family that youth will not be able to insure his own prosperity, except by insuring that of everyone else in the community. If he will wish to be happy himself, he will have to resign himself to seeing others also happy. The isolated individual does not exist except in illness—mental or physical. Society will foster individual growth towards personal fulfillment; it will be a structure brought about, maintained and reconstructed by individuals; there will be no personal fulfillment without society. There will be no world citizen, for every normal youth will depend for his health on loyalty to a delimited area of society.

Community medicine will promote health, prevent disease, treat the sick when prevention breaks down, and rehabilitate the people after they have been cured. These are highly social functions, hence we must look at medicine as a social science. Medicine will be deeply involved in the social organization of community life; and if there is any meaning in the phrase doctor-patient relation, it implies the recognition of the patient as a social being who lives in a network of relations and in the chance isolation of sickness. The patient will play a larger role in the future of medicine with health care as a right, not a privilege. The doctor's work in the future will be more and more educational and less and less curative. More and more he will deal with the physiology and psychology of his patient and less and less with his pathology. He will spend his time keeping the fit fit, rather than trying to make the unfit fit. Necessity relieves society from the embarrassment of choice. Where need speaks it demands not just food, clothing and shelter for life but food, clothing, shelter, education, employment and health care.

Screening programs for the routine examination of "health" populations will greatly improve public health by early detection and prompt treatment of the submerged moiety of symptomless disease with automated chemistry, electronic data processing and technical interpretations. They will be manned by bioengineers, freed from the older patterns of clinical thinking, borrowing from scientific management and national industry. Medicine will become a public utility. There will be hospital regionalization, health care units of coordinated medicine, health centers integrated in practice, education and research for every system of the body. The health system will provide not just for prevention and treatment of adolescent disorders but also for the continued education of those who deliver the care and for the support of research through which it is improved. All diagnostic procedures will be performed by computer systems on an assembly line. The patient's medical record from birth will be instantly available for current correlation.

Community health in developing countries will be built on the foundations of sound nutrition and safe environment. Few countries had been able to provide medical and health care for more than 20 percent of their population, so that millions were born, lived and died without any form of medical aid, other than that of the traditional practitioner. There will be moves away from the international to the supra-national approach, by examinations of the medical problems of the world as a whole, the identification of world priorities in terms of morbidity and mortality, and the organization of research units to tackle these priorities. Human development will be designed to facilitate the growth of human awareness, consciousness, self-direction and cooperation. There will be a closer relationship between youth's formal education, character, conduct and conditions of his individual and collective life.

Society will prepare youth for and expect of each adaptive responses from systemic challenges by physical and mental tasks which come at appropriate times within individual capabilities. Genetic capacity does not automatically express itself, for each capability is called forth maximally only on response to an optimum stressor level. The resulting individual happiness will oscillate between satisfaction and dissatisfaction, with a sustained sense of identity, despite continual revision of ongoing intentions as new messages from a rapidly changing world show up in their private information centers.

What performance will be within the capacities of most adolescents in the next generation? Some believe that everyone could do well and others that innate gifts are needed. The truth is between these extremes, hence the dawn of a complete revision of educational methods. Children differ in the times at which capacities mature, and in the best responses to methods for developing them. Teaching procedures for cultivating capacities below the median do great harm by wrong timing and wrong techniques. Aptitude tests will help but we may have to wait for human clonal reproduction before scientific teaching can be applied judiciously.

The primary purpose of adolescent education will be to act responsibly, to live fully, to assist others, to unravel ignorance, to remedy wrongs. The old notion that youth can learn enough in the first two decades to last him for a lifetime is as preposterous as the thought that a jet-liner can remain aloft after all its fuel has been exhausted. Learning will continue for a lifetime by technical means adapted to individual ability. Formal education will be simplified by technological advances. Human learning will become more sophisticated for ready application to youth of different backgrounds and tasks of different dimensions. Equipment proliferation from programmed texts to videotape will enable the presentation of anything to be taught more intelligibly and memorably provided the subjects take precedence over gadgetry. Computers will individualize instruction of complex topics for the most heterogeneous youth.

Education will be proportioned to the intelligence and ability of the adolescent rather than to the wealth and power of the parents. It will create finer adjustment between real life and the growing knowledge of life, make youth fit company for himself with living facts, get him out of his isolated class into one humanity. It will not be a product—diploma, job, money—but a process, never ending throughout life. It will advance meritocracy—management by the ablest—because the growth of knowledge will make ability easier to recognize. There will be democratization of professional education, decline of private inheritance and levelling of personal income differences.

Homo socialis will take over the mega-universities as service institutions for society to provide technical or professional training for youth and corrective measures for social disorders—violence, decay, pollution, dehumanization. The vital role of academic centers for the creative activities of the intellectual elite in humanities and sciences will be degraded with mass domination of all human activity. Homo individualis, creative man, will no longer be accepted for the leadership of the mass of men; Homo socialis without ivory towers' civilization will be lost in the market place.

Humanism will eventually emerge as the ideal pattern to reveal the true nature of youth and the task for him ahead, the task of shaping himself into a true man and thereby create a culture worthy of him to be transmitted to future generations. For humanism is a lasting truth; it pervades the whole process of eternal flux like a divine fire that works in each of us whether we know it or not; it is a common metaphysical faith which transcends all schisms and conflicts within; it is the core of intellectual achievement, moral action and human love.

Psychological development of youth is determined by basic drives, but the form and quality of the emerging behavior is determined by the character of environmental encounters. Mental health centers will spend less time analyzing psychological factors within the individual and more time studying the environments and the way adolescents function within them. This shift toward a greater balance of concern between intrinsic and extrinsic forces will lead to contingency management. It will be directed at the achievement of specific modifications in the behavior and environment of young people with direct participation of community members. Both will maintain and plan community facilities by continuous consultations with the adolescent's family, friends, clergy and all others conversant with his environment.

Community mental health of adolescents will thus be enhanced by using natural and contrived group interactions. An isolated youth will participate in natural groups, and disturbed youth, in contrived groups to gain better understanding of themselves and learn meaningful interaction with others under professional surveillance. Therapy will be thrust at the forces that impinge on youth from without rather than from within to make him live better rather than feel better about the way he lives. Adolescent disorders were never brought under complete control by treatment. Only through preventive measures can they be eliminated on the basis that they are not illnesses but the results of poor learning or no learning at all. Federal creation of human resources development centers will reach adolescents and their families with problems in living to prepare them for community roles.

Adequate and balanced maturation will enable youth to perform physical and mental work, respect material and spiritual values, participate in public affairs and exercise ethical ideals and aesthetic tastes. Every individual will take part in the world's work without any distinction between mental and physical performance and every youth will be required to know how machinery works, how to master it, how to assemble and improve it on the basis of a universal polytechnical training. Youth will be more humble in the face of the distractive potentials of what he can achieve and more confident of his own humanity as against robots which simulate him. The danger of the past was that men became slaves; the danger of the future is that men will become robots.

Behavior control with coercion techniques will range from the treatment of personal disorder to the reordering of human affairs at many levels. Drug administration and information control will affect individual mores and morals. Motives dictate behavior, hence disordered behavior arises from peculiarities in youth. Insight therapy will give him greater control of his aberrant behavior, liberate him from disabling symptoms and help to make his whole life more meaningful. All coordinated behavior, conscious or unconscious, will apply negative feedback. Ethical countercontrols will prevent exploitation by the use of force. But the rapid development of new control techniques will outstrip countercontrol. Psychopharmacologic agents will not be effective in brain-washing procedures.

Rebellion against the establishment will be continued by youth as it has for millennia. As a dimension of youth it actually defines him. Adolescents have a capacity but not a need for aggression but will exercise that capacity collectively unless means will be provided for youth to work towards the attainment of their aspirations. Coercion alone is ineffective because it inspires resistance rather than compliance. Youth aspire to more than physical being—to security, status, a sense of community and the right to manage their own affairs. If youth will have substantially more physical resources than status or freedom, they will use the former to gain the latter by violent means, if necessary. There is a fallacy in the assumption that all wants must be satisfied to minimize discontent. That is not a function of the discrepancy between what youth want and what they have, but between what they want and what they believe they are capable of attaining. If their means are threatened, they will revolt; if they obtain new means they will work to satisfy their wants. Youth resort to political violence with good reason. It doesn't take a majority to make a rebellion; it takes only a few determined leaders and a sound cause.

Something deeper than democracy will be required, for when leaders and followers alike realize that their effort is mental and that society's goals are their goals, they will cooperate in the vast projects with fervor. They will become willing to accept their part in whatever sacrifice is needed by sharing in the design. It is this change from drift to choice, to collective responsibility and commitment, that dominates all other changes. It is the change from the adolescent to the man. Indeed, he will be characterized by deliberation of his will to do what is best for all. Herein lies his autonomy. On such solid ground man can peer into the future that contains not only the fleeting forms of truths about the universe he has not reached, but even more important, a more penetrating understanding of himself. Yet youth doubts that current civilization has a future. It is comforting to know that such doubts existed in every generation, but our own present differs in that science is so dominant and dependable. Progress is furthered, not by conformity, but by aberration. Youth thrives on it in quest of independence not through adaptation but through daring, through obeying powerful innate drives.

> "The future of youth's past is in the future
> The future of youth's present is in the past
> The future of youth's future is in the present."

YOUTH CREDO 2000

I will recognize the need for prompt remedial action in a world beset with crisis and will work with others to formulate my beliefs and unite in a worldwide movement for the optimal development of man in harmony with nature as a vital instrument of human progress.

I will recognize the cultural uniqueness of each individual and his instinctive need to contribute to the betterment of society and will listen to the reasoned viewpoints of minorities and/or majorities in order to accept the role of emotional commitment for wisdom in action as a noble purpose in life's fulfillment.

I will recognize the inevitability of introspective suffering that results from natural disorders in man and from hazards of the physical world and will make personal sacrifices to reverse the superimposed suffering that results from man's inhumanity to man, pitilessly repeating itself from the foundation of the world—an obligation long overdue to future generations.

INDEX

Problems, learning, 87
sexual, 195
Process, developmental, 10
Processes, emotional, 136
Profile, personality, 236, 257
Programs, out-patient, 251
Promiscuity, homosexual, 204
in alienation, 185
in youth subculture, 183
Provision, psychosocial, 152
Pseudohomosexuality, 203
Pseudohypoparathyroidism, 58, 59
Pseudotransvestitism, 208
Psychotic personality, 245
Psychopathology, key to, 134
social, 171
Psychosis, 230
beginning of, 13
self-induced, 241
Psychosomatic illness, 164
Psychotherapy, for delinquents, 171
limitations of, 172
Puberty, development, female, 212
physical changes, 212
Pulmonary disease, 58
Purpose, life's, 235

Q

Qualities, mature, 281
Questioning, adolescent, 184

R

Reactions, emotional, 134
parental, 14, 15
Realism, adjustment to, 274
Reassurance, parental, 132
Reading, difficulties, 90
Reality, psychological, 117
sense of, 116
world of perceptions, 117
Reason, 94, 138
ability to, 111
Reasoning, problem-solving, 98
propositional, 109
Rebel, psychologically mature, 147
Rebellion, adolescent, 30
Regression, transitory, 121

Reidentification, psychosexual, 208
Rejection, parental, 138
Relationships, emotional, 144
heterosexual, 165
interpersonal, 122
sexual, 216, 218
social, 159
Renal disease, chronic, 58
Renunciation of needs, 168
Repression, of needs, 168
Reserves, emotional, 146
Response, coital, 225
sexual, 225
Responsibility, 153
adolescent, 132
social, 159, 165
Retardate, mental diagnostic profile, 85
environmental needs, 87
neurological defects, 89
pathologically retarded, 84
physiological retardation, 84
style of perception, 86
mental tests, 84
Retardation, mental, 82
diagnosis, 85
reading, 87
Role, adult, acceptance of, 233
choice of profession, 111
confusion, 163
Rorschach, 262

S

Sadism, 202
Satisfaction, sexual, 218
School failure, 91
alienation, 185
depressed personality, 246
Schizophrenia, drug use, 211
Self, 9
acceptance of, 167
molding of, 164
Self-awareness, 118
Self-concept, unstable, 231, 260
Self-control, social, 167
Self-direction, 123
Self-discipline, 137
Self-esteem, 120
acquisition of, 179